Nursing care

in

Maxillofacial

Surgery

The Complete Guide

ALEXANDRE CAREWELL

Table of contents

« Maxillofacial surgery: where the skilful hand restores form and function to every face. »

Chapter 1:
INTRODUCTION
TO MAXILLO-FACIAL SURGERY

Definition and background

Maxillofacial surgery, in its purest form, is the art and science of diagnosing, preventing and treating diseases, injuries and deformities of the mouth, maxilla and adjacent facial structures. It embodies a delicate fusion between dentistry and general medicine, offering holistic care that transcends mere aesthetics.

The history of this speciality dates back to ancient times. Although the techniques and instruments were rudimentary, ancient civilisations such as the Egyptians and Romans already had some understanding of oral and facial anatomy. Texts dating back several millennia bear witness to attempts to correct fractures or malocclusions.

With the Middle Ages and the Renaissance, the approach to medicine became institutionalised. Despite this, surgical practices, especially those involving the face, were often limited by a lack of precise anatomical knowledge and superstitious beliefs. It was not until the 16th and 17th centuries, with figures such as Ambroise Paré in France, that maxillofacial surgery began to stand out as a speciality.

The First World War was a major turning point. The devastating injuries suffered by soldiers required a specialised surgical approach, leading to remarkable advances in reconstructive surgery. It was against this tumultuous backdrop that maxillofacial surgery emerged as a distinct discipline, with dedicated practitioners seeking to restore not only function but also aesthetics, recognising the psychological importance of facial appearance.

Today, this speciality is not limited to post-traumatic operations. It covers a wide spectrum, from orthognathic surgery to correct malocclusions, to oncological surgery to treat tumours, to cosmetic procedures. With the advent of technology and advanced techniques, maxillofacial surgery continues to evolve, offering ever more innovative solutions to the complex challenges of the face and mouth.

Maxillofacial surgery is the fruit of a rich and complex history, born of mankind's profound need to heal, restore and beautify. It remains a constantly evolving field, reflecting man's never-ending quest for medical and aesthetic perfection.

Scope and diversity interventions

Maxillofacial surgery, with its impressive scope, extends far beyond routine operations on the teeth and gums. It encompasses a variety of procedures that reflect the complex anatomy and functions of the oral and facial region.

Start by considering congenital pathologies, such as cleft lip and palate. These malformations, present from birth, require surgery to restore form and function, enabling the child to eat, speak and breathe normally. Interventions in these cases are not just functional; they also have profound aesthetic and psychological implications for the patient and his or her family.

Orthognathic surgery treats skeletal anomalies of the jaw. Whether it's a protruding or receding jaw, or facial asymmetry, these operations aim to realign the bony structures to improve chewing, breathing, speech and, of course, the patient's appearance.

Trauma, whether caused by road accidents, falls, violence or sporting activities, can lead to fractures of the facial bones or soft tissue damage. In these situations, the intervention of a maxillo-facial surgeon is crucial to repair, realign and restore the affected area to its natural state.

Oncology also has its place in this field. Tumours, whether benign or malignant, can develop in the oral cavity, the salivary glands or other parts of the face and neck. Their excision, sometimes followed by reconstructive surgery, is essential to save lives while preserving function and aesthetics as far as possible.

Technological advances have also led to the emergence of facial cosmetic surgery, with procedures ranging from rhinoplasty and eyelid surgery to facelifts and injections.
But the diversity doesn't stop there. Think of salivary gland surgery, excision of cysts and benign tumours, or procedures to treat conditions such as sleep apnoea.

Maxillofacial surgery, with its vast scope, is truly at the crossroads between art and science. It combines an in-depth understanding of anatomy and physiology with an acute aesthetic sensitivity, all in the service of healing, well-being and the regained confidence of patients.

Technological developments and its impact on the speciality

In the medical field, technological advances have always played a pivotal role, paving the way for more accurate diagnoses, more effective treatments and a better quality of life for patients. Maxillo-facial surgery, as a speciality, is no exception to this rule and has benefited spectacularly from these advances.

Digital radiology, for example, has revolutionised the way surgeons view oral and facial anatomy. 3D imaging, such as cone-beam computed tomography (CBCT), offers a detailed view of bone and tissue structures, enabling precise surgical planning and minimising risks.

3D modelling is another innovation that has taken maxillofacial surgery by storm. Thanks to 3D printing, surgeons can create physical models of a patient's facial structures, enabling them to practise and plan procedures before even entering the operating theatre. This is particularly useful for complex or reconstructive surgery.

Telemedicine has also left its mark. With the ability to consult remotely, maxillo-facial surgeons can offer their expertise to patients in remote or inaccessible areas, breaking down geographical barriers.

The **surgical instruments** themselves have also evolved. Miniaturised and robotic instruments now allow less invasive operations, with smaller incisions, shorter recovery times and fewer post-operative complications.

The **integration of artificial intelligence** represents another revolution. With sophisticated algorithms that can analyse X-rays, predict potential complications, and even guide surgeons through certain stages of procedures, AI has proved to be a valuable ally.

However, despite all these advantages, technological change also brings challenges. Ongoing training is becoming imperative to master the new technologies. What's more, adopting these innovations can require substantial financial investment, not to mention the ethical concerns associated with, for example, telemedicine or AI.

Technological developments have undoubtedly reshaped maxillofacial surgery, propelling it into an era of efficiency, precision and almost limitless possibilities. But like all advances, it must be approached with discernment, always balancing enthusiasm for the new with an unwavering respect for patient safety and well-being.

Chapter 2:
THE ESSENTIAL ROLE OF THE NURSE

The importance of the relationship nurse-patient

In the vast world of healthcare, the relationship between nurse and patient often stands out as the central pivot around which a successful care experience revolves. In maxillofacial surgery, a speciality that touches on one of the most visible and expressive aspects of our identity, this relationship takes on an even more critical dimension.

Imagine a patient who has just undergone surgery to correct a facial deformity or remove a tumour. The emotions are intense: there may be fear, apprehension about how the operation will look afterwards, concern about pain or complications. At these vulnerable moments, the nurse often becomes the first point of contact, the person to whom the patient turns for comfort, answers and reassurance.

Trust is at the heart of this relationship. A skilled and empathetic nurse can instil a sense of security, assuring the patient that he or she is in good hands. This trust facilitates communication, encouraging the patient to ask questions, express concerns and follow post-operative advice and instructions.

Education is another essential facet. Nurses play a key role in educating patients about post-operative care, medication, signs of infection or other complications, and recovery stages. A good understanding of these elements can not only improve clinical outcomes, but also reduce patient anxiety.

Maxillofacial surgery, by touching the face, can have profound **psychological** implications. Nurses, through their proximity to and ongoing interaction with patients, are often better placed to detect signs of emotional distress, depression or anxiety. By recognising these signs, nurses can facilitate early intervention, whether in the form of psychological support, therapy or other resources.

Finally, the power of **human reassurance should not be** underestimated. A kind word, an attentive ear, or simply a reassuring presence can do wonders for a patient's emotional well-being. In a speciality where appearance, identity and function intersect, these human gestures take on particular importance.

The nurse-patient relationship in maxillofacial surgery is not limited to the simple administration of care. It is an alliance, a collaboration based on trust, education, understanding and empathy, aimed at ensuring not only the physical, but also the emotional and psychological well-being of the patient. It is this relationship that often makes the difference between an impersonal care experience and holistic healing.

The nurse as the focal point care coordination

When you enter the maze of the medical world, you quickly discover that the care process is comparable to a complex symphony. Each healthcare professional plays a unique part, essential to the harmony of the whole. At the heart of this melody is the nurse, often likened to a silent but efficient conductor, coordinating care with unparalleled dexterity.

In maxillofacial surgery, the complexity of the procedures and treatments requires close collaboration between various specialists: surgeons, anaesthetists, radiologists, physiotherapists, nutritionists and sometimes even psychologists. This is where the nurse emerges, not only as a care provider, but also as a central communicator, linking every member of the team, ensuring that every stage of treatment is orchestrated with precision.

In the pre-operative phase, it is the nurse who is often at the forefront, taking the patient's medical history, preparing the patient for the operation and communicating the relevant information to the surgical team. Later, on waking, in this delicate postoperative phase, the nurse monitors vital signs, manages pain, and ensures that the patient is recovering as expected, while keeping other healthcare professionals informed of progress or any complications.

But care coordination doesn't stop there. Nurses also play a vital role in educating patients and their families. They teach them about home care, the warning signs to look out for, and guide them through the convalescence process. The nurse's educational role strengthens the link between the patient and the medical team, ensuring continuity of care even after discharge from hospital.

Nurses are also tireless advocates for patients' needs and rights. By ensuring that each patient receives care tailored to their individual needs, listening to them and relaying their concerns to the medical team, nurses ensure that the patient's voice is always heard and respected.

In maxillofacial surgery, as in other medical fields, care coordination cannot be truly effective without the central role of the nurse. Their expertise, compassion and ability to communicate with the entire medical team make them an essential link in the care chain, ensuring harmonious, patient-centred care.

Specific skills
maxillo-facial surgery

Maxillofacial surgery, with its delicate procedures and often profound implications for patients' identity and function, requires specific skills on the part of the nurses who work in it. These skills are not limited solely to mastery of care techniques, but also encompass a panoply of knowledge, interpersonal skills and abilities specific to the specialty.

Firstly, **anatomical and physiological knowledge** of the face and jaw is essential. Understanding the complexity of the bone, muscle, vascular and nerve structures of the face enables the nurse to anticipate the patient's needs, accurately assess their condition and prevent possible complications.

In addition, **mastery of postoperative techniques specific** to maxillofacial surgery is crucial. This includes monitoring the airway, managing drains and dressings, and recognising signs of infection or other complications common in this speciality.

Maxillo-facial surgery nurses must also develop a **heightened psychological sensitivity**. Facial procedures can have a profound emotional impact on the patient, linked to questions of identity, aesthetics and self-perception. Being a good listener, showing empathy and reassuring the patient become invaluable skills in this context.

Interprofessional communication is another key skill. The nurse is often the link between the patient and the surgical team, translating the patient's concerns and needs while relaying medical directives. This ability to navigate between the patient and the various specialists involved is essential to ensure continuity and quality of care.

In addition, **educational skills** take on particular importance. Educating patients about home care, taking medication, rehabilitation exercises or even suitable diets requires appropriate teaching methods and unwavering patience.

Finally, with the constant evolution of surgical techniques and medical technologies, nurses need to have the **ability to adapt** and a desire for continuous learning. Keeping abreast of the latest advances, taking part in regular training courses and exchanging ideas with your peers are all essential steps in staying at the cutting edge of your speciality.

The unique nature and far-reaching implications of maxillofacial surgery require nurses to combine technical, interpersonal and educational skills. These skills, combined with passion and dedication, guarantee optimal, patient-centred care, reflecting the very heart of the nursing profession.

Chapter 3:
THE DAILY NEWSPAPER
IN THE MAXILLO-FACIAL DEPARTMENT

The patient's arrival: from the welcome pre-operative preparation

When a patient arrives for maxillofacial surgery, it is often with a mixture of anticipation, anxiety and hope. This pre-operative period is crucial, as it lays the foundations for a successful surgical experience and optimal recovery. It therefore requires special attention from the medical team, and the nurse plays a key role at every stage.

From the very first moment of contact, **a warm welcome** is essential. A warm smile, attentive listening and a reassuring presence can quickly ease the worries of a nervous patient. The nurse then takes the time to check the essential information: the patient's identity, the type of operation planned, medical history, current medication and, of course, to answer any questions.

Next, the **assessment phase** begins. This is the time for the nurse to carry out a full clinical assessment. This assessment includes vital measurements, a review of systems, and in particular a careful evaluation of the facial area. Any abnormalities, pain or peculiarities must be noted and communicated to the surgical team.

After the assessment, the **actual preparation** for the operation begins. This may include placing a peripheral venous line, administering pre-operative medication or applying antiseptic solutions to the area to be operated on. Throughout this preparation, the nurse takes care to inform the patient of the steps to come, reassuring and clarifying procedures to minimise anxiety.

The **educational** aspect is also essential at this stage. The nurse takes the time to explain again how the operation will be carried out, the planned post-operative care, and any signs or symptoms that may require immediate medical attention after the operation. This education phase is an opportunity for the patient to ask questions, express concerns and feel involved in their own care.

Pre-operative preparation is also the ideal time to address the **emotional and psychological aspects** of the operation. Maxillofacial operations, by affecting the face, can give rise to concerns about aesthetics and identity. By discussing fears, hopes and expectations openly, the nurse can help the patient to approach the surgery with a balanced and positive outlook.

From the initial welcome to pre-operative preparation, each stage is crucial in establishing a climate of trust, information and caring. The nurse, through his or her proximity and expertise, plays a pivotal role in ensuring that the patient approaches the operation calmly, well-informed and well-prepared.

Support during the operation

The moment of surgery represents the climax of a journey often marked by anticipation and anxiety for the patient. Although nurses are not usually the main players in this phase, their role as support staff remains crucial in ensuring the patient's well-being and the smooth running of the procedure.

Before the patient enters the operating theatre, the nurse carries out a **final check of** the essential data. This includes confirming the patient's identity, the planned procedure and the presence of all signed informed consents. This step reassures the patient that every detail has been taken into account and that he or she is in good hands.

Once in the operating theatre, the nurse helps to **position the patient** safely and comfortably. Monitoring equipment is set up: electrocardiogram, blood pressure measurement, pulse oximetry, etc. The nurse ensures that the patient is properly covered and protected, and that his or her dignity is respected at all times.

Throughout the operation, the operating theatre nurse, often referred to as **the "instrument nurse",** works closely with the surgeon. They prepare and supply the necessary instruments, anticipate the needs of the surgical team and guarantee the sterility of the operating field. Their in-depth knowledge of maxillo-facial surgery procedures enables them to act with speed and precision.

Alongside the instrument nurse, the **circulating nurse** moves freely around the operating theatre. His role is to ensure that the team has all the necessary equipment, to communicate with the outside world if necessary, and to monitor the environment to guarantee patient safety.

Even if there is no direct verbal communication with the anaesthetised patient, the **reassuring presence of the** nurse is palpable. Every action and every check is carried out with the patient's well-being in mind, ensuring their comfort and safety.

Finally, as the operation draws to a close, the nurse prepares the **patient's transfer** to the recovery room. They ensure that the patient is stable, that all drains, catheters and monitoring devices are in place, and that the transition to the postoperative phase will be seamless.

During maxillofacial surgery, the nurse remains a central pillar. Although less visible to the sleeping patient, their role is essential to the safety, efficiency and success of the procedure. Their expertise, vigilance and dedication ensure that, even in the silence and concentration of the operating theatre, the patient is accompanied and protected at all times.

Post-operative care

The post-operative period is just as delicate as the operation itself. For the patient, it is a time of vulnerability, discomfort and sometimes pain. For the nurse, it's a time of monitoring, listening and support, to ensure a healthy and rapid recovery.

As soon as the operation is over, the **transition** to the recovery room begins. The patient is transferred carefully, taking care to maintain haemodynamic stability. The recovery room nurse takes over, assessing vital signs, monitoring signs of recovery and establishing a reassuring first contact with the patient.

Once awake, one of the main concerns is **pain management**. By regularly assessing the intensity of the pain using appropriate scales, the nurse administers the painkillers prescribed, adjusts the doses if necessary and ensures that the medication is well tolerated.

Assessment of the operated area is also vital. The nurse checks for haematomas, infections or signs of post-operative complications. Drains, sutures and dressings are inspected and maintained regularly. Any changes are recorded and shared with the medical team.

Functional recovery is another key objective during this period. The nurse encourages the patient to move around, to undergo physiotherapy exercises if necessary, and to look after their nutrition and hydration, particularly after operations that may affect their ability to eat or drink normally.

Communication with the patient and their family is essential. The nurse takes the time to explain the care provided, the sensations the patient may feel, and reassures them that recovery is proceeding normally. The patient's fears, questions and needs are taken into account, creating a climate of trust and collaboration.

Before discharge, **therapeutic education is** provided. The nurse provides information on care at home, medicines to take, warning signs to look out for and how to resume daily activities. Brochures or information sheets can be given to patients as a reference.

Finally, **coordination** with other health professionals (physiotherapist, dietician, psychologist) is sometimes necessary to ensure comprehensive care, integrating all aspects of the patient's well-being.

The post-operative period in maxillofacial surgery is therefore a time of intense care, support and expertise. The nurse's holistic approach ensures not only physical healing but also the patient's emotional and psychological well-being, guaranteeing a complete and serene recovery.

Chapter 4:
TECHNIQUES
AND SPECIFIC PROTOCOLS

Asepsis procedures and sterilisation

Maxillo-facial surgery, like any other surgical speciality, requires a sterile environment to prevent post-operative infections and guarantee patient safety. Asepsis and sterilisation procedures are therefore at the heart of this discipline, representing the foundation on which the success of each operation rests.

Asepsis is first and foremost a philosophy. It involves preventing contamination by pathogenic micro-organisms. It starts long before the patient enters the operating theatre:

- **Cleaning and disinfection of premises**: The operating theatre, recovery room and adjacent areas must be thoroughly cleaned using appropriate products. Floors, surfaces and equipment are scrupulously disinfected.
- **Preparing the patient**: Before the operation, the patient is showered with an antiseptic soap. The surgical area is then shaved if necessary, and cleaned and disinfected with an appropriate antiseptic solution.
- **Dressing the medical team**: The surgeon, nurse and all other staff involved must wear sterile garments: cap, mask, gown and gloves. Dressing must follow a precise procedure to avoid contamination.

Sterilisation involves instruments and equipment that come into direct contact with the patient:

Cleaning instruments : After use, instruments are cleaned to remove any residual blood, tissue or other substances. This can be done manually or using specialised machines.

Disinfection: The instruments are then disinfected, often using ultrasonic baths to eliminate any micro-organisms present.

Sterilisation proper: Instruments are placed in autoclaves, machines that use pressurised steam to kill all forms of microbial life. Sterilisation is validated by biological and chemical indicators.

Storage: Once sterilised, instruments are kept in sterile packaging, in dry, clean places away from direct light. Their use is recorded and their expiry date monitored.

Nurses, particularly those specialising in operating theatres, are often responsible for managing and ensuring compliance with asepsis and sterilisation procedures. Their in-depth knowledge, attention to detail and commitment to patient safety make them essential players in the prevention of nosocomial infections.

In maxillofacial surgery, where operations involve sensitive areas such as the face, and are sometimes close to natural openings such as the mouth or sinuses, the importance of asepsis and sterilisation is crucial. These procedures not only ensure the success of operations, but also preserve the patient's trust in the medical team.

Care of wounds and drains

Maxillofacial surgery, involving operations on essential structures of the face and jaw, requires particular attention to post-operative wounds and drains. This care is essential not only to ensure proper healing, but also to avoid complications such as infections or haematomas.

Wound care :

- **Initial assessment**: After the operation, the nurse examines the wound for any signs of infection, excessive bleeding or suture problems. This initial assessment provides a baseline for subsequent care.
- **Cleaning**: Keeping the wound clean is essential to prevent infection. Gentle cleansing with a saline solution or mild antiseptic can be carried out, avoiding rubbing the area.
- **Dressings**: Sterile dressings are used to protect the wound from contamination and to absorb any exudate. The nurse ensures that dressings are changed as often as necessary, in accordance with the surgeon's recommendations.
- **Monitoring**: The wound is regularly assessed to ensure that it is healing properly. Any signs of infection (redness, heat, pain, pus) or problems with healing are reported immediately.

Care of drains :

- **Drain function**: Drains are often used in maxillofacial surgery to evacuate excess fluid or blood that may accumulate in the operated area. This helps to reduce the risk of haematoma and infection.
- **Flow monitoring**: The nurse regularly measures and records the amount and type of fluid drained. Sudden variations may indicate a problem.
- **Care of insertion site**: As with wounds, the drain insertion site is cleaned and protected with a sterile dressing. It is also monitored for any signs of infection or irritation.
- **Removal of the drain**: The drain is removed on the surgeon's orders, generally when the volume drained falls below a certain threshold. The nurse ensures that

this procedure is as gentle as possible for the patient, and then takes care of the site after removal.

The maxillo-facial surgery nurse plays a pivotal role in the management of wounds and drains. Thanks to their expertise, observation skills and diligence, they ensure optimal healing for the patient, while preventing post-operative complications. This responsibility requires not only technical skills, but also the ability to reassure and guide patients through every stage of their recovery.

Pain management and potential complications

Maxillofacial surgery, which involves sensitive and essential areas of the face and jaw, frequently leads to post-operative pain. In addition to pain, there are other potential complications that require specific management. The nurse is at the forefront of managing these aspects, ensuring the patient's well-being and optimum recovery.

Pain management :

Assessment: The nurse regularly assesses the patient's pain using self-assessment or observation scales, depending on the patient's ability to communicate.

Administering painkillers: Depending on the pain assessment and medical prescriptions, the nurse administers painkillers. These may range from simple analgesics to opioids for more severe pain.

Non-drug therapies: Depending on the situation, the nurse may also suggest relaxation techniques, massage or other interventions to help relieve pain.

Patient education: The nurse informs the patient about expected pain, its management and the importance of reporting any variation or increase in pain.

Potential complications :

- **Haematomas and bleeding**: Particular attention is paid to the early detection of haematomas or excessive bleeding. Any changes are reported and appropriate action taken.

- **Infections**: Despite strict aseptic measures, there is always a risk of post-operative infection. The nurse will watch for signs of infection, such as redness, warmth, swelling, pain or the presence of pus.

- **Sensory problems**: Procedures on the face can cause temporary or permanent problems with sensation. The nurse regularly assesses the patient's sensitivity and guides him/her in managing these problems.

- **Breathing difficulties**: Some surgeries, particularly those close to the respiratory tract, can lead to obstructions or breathing difficulties. The nurse is vigilant and has the necessary equipment to intervene quickly if necessary.

- **Aesthetic and psychological problems**: Maxillofacial surgery can have an impact on a patient's appearance. The nurse supports the patient in accepting their new appearance and refers them to specialists if necessary.

Managing pain and complications in maxillofacial surgery requires a combination of clinical skills, communication and empathy. The nurse's central role is to ensure the patient's comfort and safety, making the post-operative experience as gentle as possible and facilitating the path to full recovery.

Chapter 5:
EMOTIONAL CHALLENGES
AND PSYCHOLOGICAL

Understanding and managing patient anxiety

In maxillofacial surgery, an operation on such visible and sensitive parts of the body as the face and jaw is a source of anxiety for many patients. This anxiety, sometimes deeply rooted, can be exacerbated by fear of the unknown, apprehension about pain or aesthetic results. For nurses, understanding this anxiety is vital, as it plays a crucial role in preparing patients for surgery and in their post-operative recovery.

Anxiety is not just an emotional reaction; it also has an impact on the body. It can manifest itself as an increased heart rate, excessive sweating, trembling or a feeling of tightness. It is therefore vital for nurses to be able to recognise these symptoms and adapt their approach accordingly.

Establishing a relationship of trust between the nurse and the patient is the first essential step in managing anxiety. Active listening, a reassuring tone and an empathetic attitude all help to establish this trust. In addition, offering patients a space to express their fears and concerns, while providing clear and honest information about what they can expect, can considerably reduce anxiety.

Preparing the patient also plays a major role. By explaining the stages of the operation, the sensations they may experience and the healing process, nurses give patients the tools to anticipate and understand what is happening, thereby reducing their fear of the unknown.

But managing anxiety doesn't stop at communication. The use of relaxation techniques, such as deep breathing, guided meditation or therapeutic music, can also help to calm the patient before and after the operation.

Finally, it is essential to understand that each patient is unique. While some may find comfort in knowledge, others may need distraction or simple words of encouragement. The nurse, through his or her central role in the patient's care pathway, has the opportunity and responsibility to adapt his or her approach to best meet each patient's individual needs, ensuring a more serene experience and promoting optimal healing.

The resilience of the nurse dealing with difficult cases

Working in the medical field, and more specifically in maxillofacial surgery, exposes nurses to a multitude of challenges. Whether dealing with patients with complex pathologies, unexpected complications or emotionally trying situations, the nurse's ability to bounce back and persevere is sorely tested. This resilience, far from being innate, is built and cultivated throughout a career.
Difficult cases in maxillofacial surgery can give rise to a variety of emotions: sadness when faced with a young patient who has suffered an accident, frustration when surgery fails to produce the expected results, or stress when faced with a medical emergency. If left unmanaged, these emotions can lead to burnout, detachment or even medical errors. Resilience then becomes an essential skill for maintaining nurses' personal well-being while guaranteeing quality patient care.

One of the first steps in developing this resilience is awareness and acceptance. Accepting that we can't always control everything, that each patient is unique and that, despite all our skill and devotion, adverse outcomes can occur. This awareness helps to avoid the trap of self-blame.

Ongoing training and exchanges with peers also play a crucial role. By learning new techniques, sharing experiences and obtaining advice from colleagues, nurses strengthen their ability to manage complex situations. Mutual support and solidarity within a team can lessen the emotional impact of difficult cases.

Another key strategy is to develop self-care skills. This can include relaxation techniques such as meditation, or engaging in activities that bring comfort, whether sport, art or leisure. Taking time out for yourself, away from the hospital environment, can help you recharge your batteries and regain emotional balance.

Finally, for some nurses, supervision or recourse to psychological support can be beneficial, providing a safe space to express and process the emotions linked to their practice.

Resilience is not just the ability to overcome ordeals, it is also the ability to grow through them. For maxillo-facial surgery nurses, developing this quality not only ensures optimal patient care, even in the most complex cases, but also preserves their well-being and their passion for this demanding and deeply rewarding profession.

The importance of team support and debriefing

In the hustle and bustle of a maxillofacial surgery department, the importance of teamwork cannot be underestimated. Medical care is not the work of a single individual, but the coordinated result of a group of experts pooling their skills and knowledge. Team support and debriefing are two crucial elements that reinforce this cohesion and guarantee the quality of care.

Team support :
Maxillo-facial surgery procedures can be long, delicate and stressful. During these moments, the interdependence between team members is palpable. A surgeon depends on his instrumentalist, who depends on his operating assistant, who in turn depends on the recovery room nurse. This chain of interdependence forms a solid and reassuring network for the patient.

Team support is more than just technical assistance. It's also about emotional support. When faced with challenging situations or difficult decisions, knowing that you can count on a colleague's shoulder or expertise is invaluable. This sense of camaraderie and solidarity not only reduces stress, but also strengthens the sense of belonging and motivation within the team.

Debriefing:
After a procedure, especially if it has been particularly complex or if complications have arisen, it is essential to take a moment to analyse what has happened. This is where the debriefing comes in.

Debriefing is not just a tool for identifying possible errors or improvements. It is first and foremost a forum where each member of the team can express their feelings, concerns and suggestions. It provides an opportunity for collective reflection, encouraging mutual learning and strengthening team bonds.

Debriefing also has an emotional dimension. It provides an opportunity to express feelings that might otherwise remain repressed, such as frustration, sadness or incomprehension. By sharing these emotions, the team often finds a form of appeasement and resolution, thus avoiding a build-up of tension.

In maxillofacial surgery, where the stakes are both technical and human, the importance of team support and debriefing cannot be overlooked. These elements contribute not only to the effectiveness and safety of care, but also to the well-being of the professionals who, day after day, work for the health and recovery of their patients.

Chapter 6:
COLLABORATE
WITH THE SURGICAL TEAM

The dynamics of the operating team

The operating team is the essential driving force behind every successful maxillofacial surgery operation. Like a Swiss clock, each component must work in harmony to ensure efficiency, safety and quality of care. The dynamics of this team are shaped by interpersonal relationships, technical skills and well-defined roles, all orchestrated with precision.

The composition of the team :
The operating team in maxillofacial surgery is often made up of the maxillofacial surgeon, the surgical assistant, the operating theatre nurse (IBODE), the anaesthetist and the sterilisation technician. Each member has a specific function, but all must work in symbiosis.

Communication :
The key to an efficient operating team is fluid, clear communication. In surgery, where every second counts, it is imperative that instructions, requests and observations are transmitted quickly and unambiguously. A surgeon may request a specific instrument from the IBODE, who must anticipate this need. The anaesthetist must constantly inform the surgeon of the patient's condition. This communication often takes the form of words, but also gestures, glances and a mutual understanding developed through experience.

Mutual trust :
Trust is fundamental to team dynamics. The surgeon must trust his assistant to follow his movements and anticipate his needs. The IBODE must trust his colleagues to maintain a sterile environment. The anaesthetist must trust the rest of the team to report any changes in the patient's condition. This trust is built up over time, with training, consistency and repetition.

Challenges and conflict resolution :
As in any team, tensions can arise. Disagreements over technique, mistakes, misunderstandings or simply the pressure of the operating environment can lead to friction. The key is to resolve these conflicts quickly and professionally, putting the patient's well-being first. Regular debriefings and team training sessions can help to anticipate and manage these situations.

Ongoing training and development :
Maxillo-facial surgery is a constantly evolving field. New techniques, instruments and technologies emerge regularly. The operating team must be proactive in its training to stay at the cutting edge of the speciality. This thirst for learning also strengthens team cohesion, as they evolve and grow together in their expertise.

The dynamics of the maxillofacial surgery operating team are a complex dance of skills, trust and communication. When functioning at its best, it not only ensures the success of operations, but also forges lasting professional and personal bonds between its members. These bonds are the beating heart of any surgical department, propelling the team towards excellence.

Interprofessional communication

Within a hospital or clinic, inter-professional communication is the cornerstone of ensuring patient safety and effective care. In maxillofacial surgery, where procedures can be delicate, complex and multidisciplinary, clear and coordinated communication between the various healthcare professionals is crucial. This communication goes beyond the simple exchange of information: it establishes relationships of trust, facilitates decision-making and ensures smooth coordination of care.

The variety of people we talk to:
Maxillofacial surgery does not just involve the surgeon and the patient. It involves a plethora of other specialists: anaesthetists, radiologists, orthodontists, pathologists, nurses, physiotherapists, and sometimes even psychologists or social workers. Each of these professionals brings specific expertise to the table, and their harmonious collaboration is essential for holistic patient care.

The importance of a common language :
With so many experts involved, it is crucial to establish a common language to avoid misunderstandings. Medical terminology can vary from one speciality to another. Agreeing on a common vocabulary that everyone can understand is the first step towards effective interprofessional communication.

Communication tools :
Shared medical records, integrated IT systems and multidisciplinary consultation meetings (RCP) are all tools that promote fluid communication. RCPs, in particular, are key moments when all the specialists involved in a case come together to discuss, exchange ideas and draw up an optimal treatment plan.

Managing disagreements :
Disagreements are inevitable in a multidisciplinary environment. What matters, however, is how they are managed. Open, respectful and responsive communication can often resolve differences and lead to consensus. It is crucial to remember that the main objective is the patient's well-being.
Interprofessional communication training :

Recognising the importance of this skill, many institutions and professional organisations now offer specific training courses in interprofessional communication. These courses aim to strengthen interpersonal skills, raise awareness of the perspectives of other specialities and promote a culture of collaboration and mutual respect.

Interprofessional communication in maxillo-facial surgery is not a luxury, but a necessity. It ensures that every patient benefits from comprehensive care, in which all areas of expertise are mobilised and coordinated to provide the best possible care. By cultivating this culture of communication, healthcare professionals not only boost their efficiency, but also build patients' trust in the team that cares for them.

The importance of morbidity reviews and mortality

In the medical world, self-assessment and continuous learning are essential to ensure patient safety and to continually improve the quality of care. Morbidity and mortality reviews (MMRs) play a central role in this respect, particularly in specialities as sensitive as maxillofacial surgery.

What is a RMM?

A morbidity and mortality review is a structured meeting at which healthcare professionals examine cases where patients have suffered complications (morbidity) or died (mortality). The aim is not to assign blame, but to understand the underlying causes, learn from these events and make improvements.

Learning from mistakes :

Even in the most competent hands, medicine is never risk-free. Complications can arise for a variety of reasons, whether it's an unforeseen factor in the patient, a clinical decision or a systemic flaw. By analysing these cases in depth, teams can identify areas for improvement, whether in their techniques, procedures or communication.

Promoting a safety culture :

MMRs play an essential role in promoting a culture of safety within medical establishments. By encouraging transparency, honesty and the sharing of experiences, they help to destigmatise medical error. Rather than hiding or denying errors, professionals are encouraged to examine them constructively.

Improving procedures and protocols :

Thanks to the lessons learned from MMRs, hospitals can implement concrete changes to improve patient safety. Whether it's adopting new technologies, modifying surgical protocols or reinforcing continuing education, the actions resulting from these reviews have a direct impact on the quality of care.

Strengthening team cohesion :

MMRs can also strengthen cohesion and collaboration within medical teams. By bringing together professionals from different disciplines to discuss complex challenges openly, they create a space of mutual trust and respect.

Morbidity and mortality reviews are much more than just an administrative formality. They reflect a deep commitment to clinical excellence and patient safety. In maxillofacial surgery, where the margins for error are slim and the consequences potentially serious, their role is all the more crucial. They are a pillar of continuous improvement, ensuring that every intervention, every decision, is informed by the lessons of the past.

Chapter 7:
ANATOMY AND PHYSIOLOGY
THE MAXILLOFACIAL REGION

Bone structures

Exploring maxillofacial surgery requires a thorough understanding of the anatomy of the face, in particular the bony structures. These bones form the framework of the face, support the soft tissues and play a crucial role in functions such as chewing, speaking and breathing.

1. The frontal bone :
Located in the upper part of the face, the frontal bone forms the forehead and the upper part of the orbits. It plays an essential role in protecting the brain and in facial expression.

2. Maxillary bones (upper jaw) :
These are the upper jawbones that support the upper teeth and form the hard palate. They play an essential role in chewing and speaking.

3. The mandibular bone (lower jaw) :
It is the largest bone in the face, mobile and articulated with the skull. It supports the lower teeth and is essential for chewing, speaking and opening/closing the mouth.

4. The zygomatic bones (or malar bones) :
Located on either side of the face, they form the cheekbones and are involved in the formation of the eye socket.

5. The nasal bone :
These are the small bones at the base of the nose that contribute to the shape and structure of this part of the face.

6. The palatine bones :

Located behind the jawbones, they form the posterior part of the hard palate and the floor of the nasal cavity.

7. The lacrimal bones :

These small bones, located inside the orbit, are in contact with the tear duct.

8. The vomer bone :

It is a thin, flat bone that forms the back of the nasal septum.

9. The ethmoid and sphenoid bones :

These complex bones are found at the base of the skull, playing an essential role in the formation of the orbits and the separation of the nasal cavity from the brain.

10. The lower nasal concha :

It is responsible for circulating and humidifying the air inhaled through the nostrils.

Surgical implications :

Knowledge of bone structures is vital for the maxillo-facial surgeon. Whether for reconstruction after trauma, correction of congenital malformations or cosmetic procedures, each bone of the face has its own anatomical and functional particularities. Surgical techniques, approaches and procedures vary depending on the bone involved and the adjacent structures.

Maxillofacial surgery is a highly precise field, requiring extensive anatomical expertise. The facial bone structures, with their complexity and interrelation, are at the heart of this speciality, guaranteeing facial functionality and aesthetics.

Vascularisation and innervation

Maxillofacial surgery, with its emphasis on the restoration and repair of facial structures, requires an in-depth knowledge of the vascularisation and innervation of this region. This is crucial not only to the functional success of operations, but also to minimising complications and ensuring optimal recovery.

Vascularisation :
Blood circulation in the face is mainly provided by branches of the external carotid artery.

- **Facial artery**: This follows a tortuous path across the face, supplying the lips, nose and eyelids.
- **Maxillary artery: This** deeper artery supplies blood to the teeth, sinuses, palate and part of the masticatory muscles.
- **Superficial temporal artery**: Rises towards the scalp, supplying the temple and anterior scalp.
- **Angular artery**: This is the continuation of the facial artery and vascularises the lateral part of the nose and part of the orbit.

Venous return is ensured by veins accompanying these arteries, draining ultimately into the internal and external jugular veins.

Innervation :
The face is mainly innervated by branches of the trigeminal nerve (V), which is the fifth cranial nerve.

- **Ophthalmic branch (V1)**: It innervates the upper eyelid, the forehead and the anterior part of the scalp.
- **Maxillary branch (V2)**: This branch innervates the lower eyelid, cheek, nose, upper lip and palate.
- **Mandibular branch (V3)**: Responsible for the innervation of the lower jaw, including the lower lip, as well as certain masticatory muscles.

Other cranial nerves also play a role, such as the facial nerve (VII) for the muscles of facial expression, and the glossopharyngeal (IX) and vagus (X) nerves for more posterior regions of the mouth and throat.

Surgical implications :
Precise knowledge of vascularisation and innervation is essential to avoid complications, particularly haemorrhage and sensory or motor deficits. It also enables the surgeon to perform vascular and nerve anastomoses during complex reconstructions, ensuring optimal viability and function of the transplanted or repaired tissue.

In addition, with advances in technology, maxillofacial surgery can now use advanced imaging techniques to map these structures pre-operatively, offering better surgical planning.

The art of maxillofacial surgery lies as much in in-depth theoretical knowledge of anatomical structures as in technical skill. The vascularisation and innervation of the face are key elements in this knowledge, guaranteeing safe and effective operations.

Tissue characteristics : muscles, skin and mucous membranes

Maxillofacial surgery involves more than just bones and joints; it interacts profoundly with the various tissues that cover and support these structures. An intimate understanding of tissue particularities is essential to ensure the aesthetic and functional success of procedures.

1. Muscles:
The face is an orchestra of muscles that give expression, emotion and function. They are so complex that each muscle has a precise role.

> **Muscles of mastication**: These include the masseter, temporalis and pterygoids (lateral and medial). They are essential for opening, closing and moving the jaw.
> **Facial expression muscles**: These muscles, such as the orbicularis orbicularis, the zygomaticus major and

the frontal, allow a range of emotional expressions, from surprise to smiling.
Surgery on these muscles requires extreme delicacy to avoid paralysis or post-operative asymmetry.

2. Skin:

The skin on the face is unique. It is fine, has a rich blood supply and is often exposed to the sun.

> **Elasticity and healing**: Facial skin is elastic and has an impressive healing capacity. However, it is essential to make precise incisions to ensure minimal and discreet scarring.

> **Regional variations**: The skin varies considerably between the forehead, eyelids, cheeks and chin in terms of thickness and elasticity.

3. Mucous membranes:

Mucous membranes are the inner linings of the mouth, cheeks and nose. They are moist, sensitive and play a crucial role in sensation and function.

> **Healing**: Mucous membranes have a rapid healing capacity, but can be prone to infection if not properly cared for.

> **Sensitivity**: They are richly innervated, making surgical procedures in these areas particularly delicate.

Surgical implications:

When working on these tissues, surgeons must take account of their vascularisation, innervation and unique properties to minimise scarring, preserve sensation and ensure optimal recovery and function.

For example, when carrying out facelifts or aesthetic procedures, it is vital to understand how the skin and muscles interact to achieve a natural result. Similarly, in oral surgery, understanding the mucous membranes is essential to ensure correct healing and prevent complications.

The soft tissues of the face, although often overshadowed by the attention paid to bony structures in maxillofacial surgery, play an equally vital role. Their complexity and interdependence require particular expertise and attention to ensure the best surgical results.

Chapter 8:
TOOLS AND TECHNOLOGIES IN MAXILLO-FACIAL SURGERY

Common surgical instruments and their use

Maxillo-facial surgery, like other surgical specialities, requires a specific range of instruments to perform precise and specialised procedures. These instruments are designed to adapt to the complex and delicate anatomical structures of the face and jaw. Here are some of the most commonly used instruments and their specific role:

1. Dissection and exposure instruments :
   - **Scalpels: These are** sharp blades used to make precise incisions. They can have different designs and blade sizes adapted to different areas of the face.
   - **Surgical scissors**: Used to cut tissue. Scissors can be straight or curved and are suitable for fine or coarse dissection.
   - **Retractors**: Instruments for retracting tissue and providing better visibility during surgery. Some are self-retaining, while others require manual handling.
2. Gripping and fastening tools :
   - **Dissecting forceps**: These are used to grasp and gently stabilise tissues during dissection or suturing.
   - **Haemostatic forceps**: These are used to grasp and clamp blood vessels, stopping bleeding. Common examples include Kelly and Crile forceps.
3. Bone instruments :
   - **Osteotomes:** Sharp instruments for cutting or shaping bone.
   - **Rodents:** Useful for removing or trimming pieces of bone.

Surgical hammers: Used with osteotomes to apply precise forces when cutting bone.
4. Suture instruments :
   Needle holders: These hold the needles firmly when suturing tissue.
   Tweezers: Used to manoeuvre and position sutures when placing or removing them.
5. Specialised instruments :
   Tear probe: A fine instrument for exploring and clearing the tear ducts.
   Oscillating saw: Used for osteotomies, particularly during orthognathic surgery.
   Surgical drills: To prepare sites for dental implants or for other operations requiring holes in the bone.
6. Suction :
   Suction cannulas: These are used to remove fluids, such as blood or saliva, to keep the operating field clean and clear.

Maxillofacial surgery requires a combination of instruments, ranging from basic tools to highly specialised devices. Each instrument is designed to optimise the efficiency and safety of operations. Perfect mastery of these tools, combined with a thorough understanding of facial anatomy, is essential to ensure the best surgical results.

Imaging technology : radiography, scanner, MRI

Maxillofacial surgery, being a speciality focused on the complex anatomy of the face, skull and jaw, relies heavily on medical imaging for the diagnosis, planning and evaluation of operations. Let's take a closer look at the main imaging modalities used and their specific features in this field:

1. Radiography :
    Dental Panoramic: This is a radiographic technique that provides a wide view of the upper and lower jaw. It is commonly used to assess the teeth, jaws and associated pathologies.
    Teleradiography of the skull: A specialised technique for visualising the skull from the side. It is often used in orthodontics and orthognathic surgery to assess the relationship between the skull, jaw and teeth.
2. Computed tomography (CT or Scanner) :
    Cross-sectional representation: The scanner uses X-rays to produce sliced images of the body. In maxillofacial surgery, it can provide precise details of the bones of the face and skull.
    3D reconstruction: Thanks to modern technology, CT images can be reconstructed to provide a three-dimensional view. This is particularly useful for surgical planning, such as trauma or reconstructive surgery.
    Cone Beam CT (CBCT): A variant of the conventional CT scanner, CBCT is specially designed for craniofacial imaging. It offers high-resolution detail with a reduced radiation dose, making it ideal for dental and maxillofacial procedures.
3. Magnetic Resonance Imaging (MRI) :
    Soft tissue and vascularisation: Unlike CT, which is excellent for bone, MRI excels at visualising soft tissue. It is often used to assess masses, tumours or infections in the soft tissues of the face and oral cavity.
    Radiation-free imaging: MRI uses magnetic fields, not radiation, making it ideal for repeated assessments or for radiation-sensitive patients.
    Contrast: The use of contrast agents in MRI can help to highlight certain pathologies or vascular structures.

Imaging plays a pivotal role in maxillofacial surgery. Whether to diagnose pathology, plan an operation or monitor post-operative recovery, each imaging modality offers specific advantages. The choice between an X-ray, a CT scan or an MRI will depend on the clinical question to be answered and the anatomical details required for assessment. Thanks to these technologies, surgeons can operate with greater precision, improving patient outcomes.

Recent innovations: robot-assisted surgery, 3D reconstruction techniques

The world of maxillofacial surgery is constantly evolving, with new technologies and techniques emerging every year. Among these innovations, robot-assisted surgery and 3D reconstruction techniques have particularly stood out in recent years.

1. Robot-assisted surgery :
   - **Greater precision**: Surgical robots offer exceptional precision, reducing the risk of human error. This is particularly useful in delicate areas of the face, where a minimum margin of error is crucial.
   - **Less invasive**: Incisions are often smaller with robotic surgery, leading to reduced scarring and a faster recovery time for the patient.
   - **Improved accessibility**: In hard-to-reach areas, the robot's articulated arms can reach with an ease that the human hand cannot always match.
   - **Training and simulation**: Robotic platforms also allow surgeons to train on simulations before performing real operations, increasing their skill and confidence.

2. 3D reconstruction techniques :

   Surgical planning: With 3D reconstruction software, surgeons can visualise their patient's anatomical structure in three dimensions. This enables them to plan and simulate their operations with unrivalled precision.

   3D printing: By combining 3D reconstruction with 3D printing, it is possible to create tailor-made implants or surgical guides for each patient. Whether replacing lost bone or guiding an incision, this technology offers unprecedented customisation.

   Visualisation during the operation: Some advanced systems allow surgeons to superimpose 3D images on the operating field during the operation, serving as a guide in real time.

   Training and education: 3D models can also be used to train students and young surgeons, giving them a realistic representation of the challenges they will face in the operating theatre.

Technological innovations are transforming maxillofacial surgery, offering both surgeons and patients considerable benefits. Robot-assisted surgery promises greater precision and safety, while 3D reconstruction techniques open the door to unprecedented customisation and surgical planning. Together, these innovations push back the boundaries of what is possible in the field and promise more effective, safer and more personalised care for patients.

Chapter 9:
COMMON PATHOLOGIES
AND ASSOCIATED TREATMENTS

Tumours and lesions
the maxillofacial region

The maxillofacial region is an anatomically complex area encompassing the jaw, mouth, face and parts of the skull. The presence of a multitude of tissues - bony, dental, mucosal, glandular, nervous and vascular - makes this region susceptible to a variety of tumours and lesions, both benign and malignant.

1. Benign tumours :
   Odontogenic cysts: Often associated with impacted teeth or dental infections, these cysts can cause bone expansion and often require surgery.
   Osteomas: Benign bone tumours that can develop on the jaw or other facial bones.
   Fibromas: Tumours of connective tissue which may occur in the gums or mucous membranes.
   Pleomorphic adenomas: Tumours of the salivary glands, usually the parotid gland, which are usually benign.
2. Malignant tumours :
   Squamous cell carcinomas: The most common malignant tumours of the oral cavity, generally associated with risk factors such as smoking, alcohol consumption or exposure to the human papillomavirus (HPV).
   Adenocarcinomas: Malignant tumours that develop from glands, such as the salivary glands.
   Sarcomas: Malignant tumours of soft tissue or bone, rare but potentially aggressive.

Malignant melanomas: Although more common on the skin, these pigment cell tumours can sometimes occur in the oral region.

3. Pre-cancerous lesions :

Leukoplakia: A non-displaceable white lesion on the oral mucosa, a proportion of which may develop into cancer.

Erythroplasia: A red, often velvety lesion with a high risk of malignant transformation.

4. Causes and risk factors :

In addition to genetic factors, exposure to tobacco, alcohol, HPV and poor oral hygiene can increase the likelihood of developing tumours in this area.

5. Diagnosis and treatment :

Diagnosis is usually made using a biopsy, followed by medical imaging (X-rays, CT scan, MRI) to assess the extent of the tumour. Treatment may include surgery, radiotherapy, chemotherapy or a combination of these, depending on the nature and location of the tumour.

Tumours and lesions of the maxillofacial region represent a varied spectrum of pathologies, from benign to malignant. Early management by a multidisciplinary team is essential to ensure the best possible prognosis for the patient. Knowledge of the signs and symptoms by healthcare professionals, as well as the public, is crucial for early diagnosis and successful intervention.

Trauma and fractures

As the most prominent part of the human anatomy, the face is often the first to be exposed to impact or trauma. Whether caused by road accidents, falls, acts of violence or sporting accidents, maxillofacial trauma can vary in severity, from minor abrasions to complex fractures.

1. Common types of maxillofacial fractures :
    Fracture of the orbital floor: This can lead to the eye sinking in and requires surgery to preserve vision and aesthetics.
    Maxillary fracture: Impacts the upper jaw, and can influence dental alignment.
    Fracture of the mandible: The lower jaw is one of the most frequently fractured bones in the face.
    Fractures of the zygomatic complex: These involve the prominent bones of the cheekbones.
    Nose fractures: Often associated with sports injuries or altercations.
2. Symptoms and signs :
    Swelling and bruising
    Pain, particularly when chewing
    Numbness due to nerve damage
    Malocclusion or change in dental alignment
    Limitation of mouth opening
    Visible or palpable deformity
3. Diagnosis :
Imaging, such as X-ray, CT scan or MRI, is essential to assess the extent and exact nature of the fracture. A thorough clinical examination is also crucial.
4. Processing :
    Surgery: In cases of displaced or complex fractures, surgery is often required to realign and fix the bones. This may involve the use of plates, screws or wires.
    Conservative treatment: For non-displaced fractures, rest, painkillers and sometimes immobilisation may suffice.
    Rehabilitation: Physiotherapy may be necessary to regain full function of the jaw, particularly in cases of persistent stiffness or pain.
5. Prevention :
Raising awareness of the use of protective equipment, such as helmets and mouthguards, during sporting

activities is essential. Promoting road safety and preventing violence are also crucial.

Trauma and fractures of the maxillofacial region are not only painful, but can have lasting aesthetic and functional consequences. Prompt and appropriate treatment is essential to optimise results and prevent complications. Raising awareness of the need to prevent these injuries is also crucial to reducing their incidence.

Congenital malformations and surgical corrections

Congenital malformations of the maxillofacial region are anomalies present from birth, resulting from a disturbance in embryonic development. These malformations can have aesthetic, functional and psychological consequences. Surgery plays a key role in correcting these anomalies to improve patients' quality of life.

1. Common types of congenital malformations :
   - **Cleft lip and/or palate: These are** divisions or openings in the upper lip and/or palate. They may be unilateral or bilateral.
   - **Micrognathia or retrognathia:** A small or abnormally positioned mandible.
   - **Haemangiomas:** Benign tumours consisting of abnormal blood vessels that can develop on the skin or inside the mouth.
   - **Craniofacial syndromes**: such as Crouzon syndrome or Apert syndrome, which involve abnormalities in the development of the skull and face.
2. Surgical management :
   - **Cleft lip and palate correction**: These operations are often performed in several stages to repair the defect

and improve function and aesthetics. The first surgery is usually performed during infancy.

- **Mandibular advancement**: In cases of severe micrognathia, an operation may be required to advance the mandible, thereby improving respiratory function and dental occlusion.
- **Resection of haemangiomas**: If a haemangioma is large or poses a risk to vital structures, surgery may be necessary.
- **Craniofacial surgery**: For craniofacial syndromes, complex surgery is often required to reshape the skull and face, improving brain function, breathing and appearance.

3. The importance of multidisciplinary management :

The correction of congenital maxillofacial malformations often requires the intervention of a team of specialists, including maxillofacial surgeons, orthodontists, paediatricians, speech therapists, psychologists and other health professionals.

4. Psychosocial considerations :

Children born with facial malformations can face psychological challenges, such as problems with self-esteem and the risk of stigmatisation. Psychological care is essential to support these children and their families.

Congenital malformations of the maxillofacial region can present considerable challenges for children and their families. Fortunately, thanks to advances in surgery and multidisciplinary management, many children can look forward to a significant improvement in their appearance and function. The key is early intervention, careful planning and long-term follow-up to ensure the best possible results.

Chapter 10:
COSMETIC SURGERY
MAXILLO-FACIAL

Pre-operative assessment
and patient expectations

The pre-operative assessment is a crucial stage before any surgical operation. It not only ensures patient safety, but also aligns patient expectations with the actual possibilities offered by surgery. In maxillofacial surgery, given the aesthetic and functional impact of operations, this stage is of particular importance.

1. Clinical assessment :
    Physical examination: This involves a detailed assessment of the facial area, including the skin, bones, teeth and soft tissues.
    Medical history: Understanding underlying illnesses, allergies, current medication or previous surgery is crucial to avoiding complications.
    Dental examination and occlusion: An assessment of dental alignment and bite may be necessary, especially for orthognathic procedures.
2. Imaging and other tests :
    X-rays, CT scans, MRI: These images provide a detailed view of the internal structures, helping the surgeon to plan the operation.
    Dental models: In some cases, dental casts can be made to study occlusion.
    Blood tests: These may be required to assess overall health and check aspects such as coagulation.

3. Discussion of expectations :
   Assessing the patient's wishes: It is essential to understand what the patient hopes to achieve after surgery.
   Matching medical reality: Sometimes, the patient's expectations may not be realistic. The surgeon must then clarify what is medically possible.
   Risks and benefits: Every operation has its benefits and risks. The patient must be fully informed in order to give informed consent.
4. Psychological preparation :
   Emotional impact: Maxillo-facial surgery can have a significant impact on self-esteem. A psychological assessment may sometimes be necessary.
   Support: Encouraging patients to talk to their families or join support groups can help them prepare emotionally for the procedure.

The pre-operative assessment is much more than a simple medical check-up. It is the bridge between the patient's wishes and concerns and the medical reality of what surgery can offer. In maxillofacial surgery, where the outcome has a profound impact on appearance and function, careful assessment and open communication are essential to ensure patient satisfaction and the success of the operation.

Common surgical techniques: rhinoplasty, facelift, genioplasty

Aesthetic and reconstructive surgery of the maxillofacial region encompasses a variety of procedures, each with its own specific techniques and objectives. Three of the most common procedures in this area are rhinoplasty, facelift and genioplasty.

65

1. Rhinoplasty :
This is a surgical procedure designed to change the shape and/or function of the nose.

  Types :
  Aesthetic rhinoplasty: Modifies the shape of the nose for cosmetic reasons.
  Functional rhinoplasty: Corrects structural abnormalities that can cause breathing problems.

  Techniques:
  Open approach: Incision at the base of the nose allowing direct visibility.
  Closed approach: Incisions inside the nostrils with no visible external incision.

  Results: In addition to aesthetic improvements, can improve breathing when septum deviations or other internal anomalies are corrected.

2. Facelift (or cervico-facial lift) :
This surgery aims to rejuvenate the face by correcting tissue laxity.

  Target areas :
  Forehead lift: Forehead and eyebrows.
  Mid-face lift: Cheeks and periocular region.
  Lower face and neck lift: Jaw, neck and area under the chin.

  Techniques:
  Strategically placed incisions around the hairline, ears and/or neck.
  Redraping of the underlying tissues and removal of excess skin.

  Results: Rejuvenated appearance, more defined contours and reduction in fine lines and wrinkles.

3. Genioplasty :
This is an operation that changes the shape of the chin.

  Types :
  Advancement: For a receding chin.
  Recession: For a prominent chin.

  Techniques:

Incision inside the mouth or under the chin.
The chin is either advanced with fixation using plates and screws, or reshaped by removing part of the bone.

Results: A chin that is better proportioned to the rest of the face, improving facial balance.

Whether for aesthetic or functional reasons, maxillofacial surgery offers a range of procedures that can have a profound impact on a person's appearance and quality of life. As with all procedures, a thorough consultation with a qualified surgeon is essential to determine the best approach for each individual patient.

Post-operative care and managing complications

The post-operative period plays an essential role in the recovery and success of a maxillofacial operation. During this phase, the nurse works closely with the medical team to minimise the risk of complications, relieve pain and facilitate the patient's convalescence.

1. Post-operative care :

Immediate monitoring: After the operation, the patient is generally transferred to the recovery room, where vital functions are closely monitored.

Pain management: Analgesics, often combined with anti-inflammatories, are administered to control pain.

Wound care: Stitches, dressings and drains are inspected regularly for signs of infection or bleeding.

Food and hydration: Depending on the nature of the operation, liquid or soft food may be recommended. Good hydration is also essential.

Mobilisation: Encouraging patients to mobilise gradually helps prevent complications such as thrombosis.

Advice on returning home: Recommendations on home care, taking medication, diet and activities to be avoided are provided to patients and their families.

2. Management of complications :

Haemorrhage: Excessive post-operative bleeding requires rapid intervention to locate and control the source.

Infection: Signs of infection, such as redness, swelling or pus, should be treated immediately with antibiotics.

Sensory disorders: Numbness or tingling may occur. If these symptoms persist, a neurological assessment may be necessary.

Abnormal scarring: Scar hypertrophy or keloids may require further treatment, such as steroid injections or reconstructive surgery.

Respiratory difficulties: Following certain types of surgery, there may be a risk of airway obstruction requiring urgent intervention.

Dehydration: Insufficient fluid intake can lead to dehydration, especially if the patient has difficulty eating or drinking after the operation.

The post-operative period in maxillofacial surgery is as critical as the operation itself. Careful monitoring, appropriate management and open communication with the patient are essential to ensure an uncomplicated recovery. If even the slightest abnormality is detected, prompt and appropriate intervention can prevent more serious complications, thereby guaranteeing the long-term success of the surgery.

Chapter 11:
ETHICS AND LEGALITY
IN MAXILLO-FACIAL SURGERY

Patients' rights and duties

When a person becomes a patient in a medical environment, they acquire a set of rights as well as responsibilities. These rights and duties are designed to guarantee respectful and effective care, while involving patients in their own care process.

1. Patients' rights :

Right to information: Patients have the right to be informed in a clear and comprehensible manner about their state of health, the proposed treatments, their benefits and risks, and possible alternatives.

Informed consent: No intervention or treatment can be carried out without the patient's free and informed consent, unless it is a life-threatening emergency.

Right to confidentiality: All information concerning the patient, including his/her identity, is confidential. It may only be shared with the medical staff involved in the care or with persons authorised by the patient.

Right of access to medical records: Patients have the right to consult and obtain a copy of their medical records.

Right to respect and dignity: Patients must be treated with respect, regardless of their age, sex, origin or any other characteristic.

Right to non-discrimination: Care must not vary according to discriminatory criteria.

Right to refuse treatment: A patient may refuse treatment or an intervention after understanding the consequences.

- **Right to continuity of care**: Patients have the right to receive continuous, coordinated care appropriate to their needs.

2. The patient's duties :
- **Honesty and transparency**: To ensure effective care, patients must provide complete and accurate information about their state of health, history, current treatments and any other relevant information.
- **Respect for medical staff**: Respecting healthcare professionals, hospital staff and other patients is essential to the smooth running of the medical establishment.
- **Compliance with rules and procedures**: This includes compliance with visiting times, health and safety procedures, etc.
- **Active participation in care**: Although patients have the right to refuse treatment, if they consent to it, they must actively participate in their own healing process.
- **Financial responsibility**: Patients must meet their financial obligations to the medical establishment or care providers.

The relationship between patient and healthcare professional is based on mutual trust. Patients' rights guarantee respectful, patient-centred medical care, while their duties ensure optimal collaboration for the benefit of their health. In the delicate field of maxillofacial surgery, this collaboration is all the more crucial to guarantee optimal results.

Informed consent and decision-making capacity

At the heart of the medical relationship is the fundamental principle of respect for patient autonomy. Two key concepts flow from this: informed consent and decision-making capacity. These concepts, although intimately linked, are distinct and play a vital role, particularly in specialities such as maxillofacial surgery, where operations can have major aesthetic and functional consequences.

1. Informed consent :

Definition: Informed consent is the agreement freely given by a patient to a medical intervention after having received all the information necessary to make an informed decision.

Elements of informed consent :

Information: The healthcare professional must provide the patient with detailed information on the nature of the procedure, the expected benefits, the possible risks, the alternatives available, and the consequences of not undergoing treatment.

Understanding: The patient must have the cognitive and emotional capacity to understand the information provided.

Will: The patient's decision must be taken without coercion or external influence.

Documentation: Informed consent is often formalised in a written document signed by the patient. Although this document is essential, the informed consent process is much more than a simple administrative formality.

2. Decision-making capacity :

Definition: This is an individual's ability to make decisions about their medical care. It is determined by the patient's ability to understand, appreciate, reason and express a preference concerning a medical decision.

Capacity assessment :

Comprehension: Is the patient able to understand the information provided by the healthcare professional?

- **Assessment**: Is the patient able to assess the relevance of the information to his/her situation?
- **Reasoning** : Can they weigh up the pros and cons of different options?
- **Expression of choice**: Can they clearly express a preference?
- **Limits to decision-making capacity**: If a patient is deemed incapable of making an informed decision, the decision may be taken by a legal representative or guardian. However, it is crucial to always seek to involve the patient as much as possible.

In maxillofacial surgery, respect for patient autonomy is of paramount importance. The concepts of informed consent and decision-making capacity help to ensure that each operation is not only medically justified, but also in line with the patient's wishes and values. In a field where the consequences of surgery can profoundly affect a person's life, it is essential to establish transparent and respectful communication between the patient and the medical team.

Managing common ethical dilemmas

In medical practice, ethical dilemmas arise when fundamental moral principles come into conflict. In maxillofacial surgery, given the intimate nature of procedures involving the face - the reflection of our identity - these dilemmas can be particularly intense.

1. Autonomy vs. benevolence :
- **Dilemma**: A patient wants cosmetic surgery to look like a celebrity, but the surgeon believes that the result will not be natural or beneficial in the long term.
- **Management**: Engaging in an open dialogue with the patient, clarifying their motivations, and educating

them about the risks and benefits. While respecting the patient's autonomy, the surgeon must ensure that the patient makes an informed decision.

2. Non-maleficence vs. benevolence :

Dilemma: A patient needs a potentially painful operation to restore jaw function, but is anxious and reluctant.

Management: Although the surgeon wishes to do what is beneficial (beneficence), he must also ensure that he does not cause harm (non-maleficence). One approach might be to explore alternative or complementary methods of managing the patient's pain and anxiety.

3. Justice vs. Autonomy :

Dilemma: An expensive procedure is available, but the healthcare system has limited resources. Who should benefit?

Management: The medical team must assess the usefulness and necessity of the intervention for each patient. Decisions should be based on equitable clinical criteria rather than ability to pay or social status.

4. Confidentiality vs:

Dilemma: A teenager wants an operation without informing his parents.

Management: In many jurisdictions, parental consent is required for interventions on minors. However, if the adolescent is deemed mature, an exception may be considered. The surgeon must balance the teenager's right to confidentiality with the principle of beneficence.

5. Aesthetic vs. functional results :

Dilemma: Intervention can restore function but alter appearance, or vice versa.

Management: Transparent communication is essential. The patient must be fully informed of the advantages and disadvantages of each option and actively participate in the decision.

When faced with ethical dilemmas, there is often no single "correct" answer. In maxillofacial surgery, as in other medical fields, the most important thing is to engage in a process of ethical reflection, to actively involve the patient and, where possible, to consult ethics committees or colleagues for additional perspectives. The key lies in the delicate balance between respecting patient autonomy and acting in the patient's best interests.

Chapter 12:
COMMUNICATION
WITH THE PATIENT AND FAMILY

Effective communication techniques

Communication is an essential element of the doctor-patient relationship, particularly in a speciality such as maxillofacial surgery where the aesthetic, functional and emotional implications of operations are closely intertwined. Clear, empathetic and effective communication can improve patient satisfaction, build trust and enhance clinical outcomes.

1. Active listening :
   Understand before you are understood: Pay full attention to the patient, without interruption. This allows you to fully understand their concerns.
   Reflection: Repeat what you have heard to confirm your understanding.
2. Non-verbal language :
   Eye contact: This establishes a bond of trust and shows that you are committed to the conversation.
   Open gestures: Avoid crossing your arms or sitting back. Adopt an open posture, leaning towards the patient.
3. Ask open-ended questions :
   Encourage the patient to talk in detail by asking questions such as: "Can you tell me more about...?" instead of closed questions requiring "yes" or "no" answers.
4. Validating the patient's feelings :
   Acknowledge and validate the patient's emotions, for example: "I can understand why you feel that way...".

5. Avoid medical words :
   Use simple, clear language to explain procedures, diagnoses and treatments. Make sure the patient understands each step.
6. Using the "Teach-Back" :
   After giving information, ask the patient to repeat back to you what they have understood. This is one way of ensuring that the information has been correctly assimilated.
7. Provide written resources :
   Give the patient brochures or information sheets to supplement verbal discussions.
8. Encourage questions :
   Make sure the patient feels comfortable asking questions. This can clarify any misunderstandings and reinforce understanding.
9. Establishing a partnership :
   Think of the patient as a partner in care decisions, actively involving them in the decision-making process.
10. Show empathy :
   Putting yourself in the patient's shoes, acknowledging their emotions and showing understanding can greatly improve the quality of communication.

Communication techniques are not simply tools for transmitting information; they are the foundation of the doctor-patient relationship. In maxillofacial surgery, where procedures can have a profound impact on identity and self-esteem, effective communication is crucial. By investing time and energy in communication training, professionals can improve not only the patient experience, but also clinical outcomes.

Dealing with bad news and unfulfilled expectations

In maxillofacial surgery, as in many other medical fields, there may be times when the professional is faced with the delicate task of communicating disappointing or unexpected news to a patient. This may be due to complications, unwanted results or unexpected discoveries. Handling these situations with compassion, tact and clarity is essential to maintaining trust and facilitating patient understanding.

1. Preparation :
    Anticipate reactions: Try to predict the patient's emotions and questions so that you are prepared to respond.
    Choose the right environment: Make sure you have a quiet, private place to talk, free from distractions.

2. Using the SPIKES model :
This model is commonly used to deliver bad news in the medical field:
    S - Setting: Make sure the location is appropriate and that you won't be interrupted.
    P - Perception (Perception): Ask the patient what they already know or what they perceive about the situation.
    I - Invitation (Invitation) : Ask permission to share the news, e.g. "Would you like me to give you more details about the results?"
    K - Knowledge: Give information clearly and avoid medical jargon. Be direct but empathetic.
    E - Emotions (Emotions): Acknowledge and validate the patient's emotions. "I understand that this may be disappointing for you."
    S - Strategy: Propose a strategy or action plan for the future.

3. Be honest but empathetic:
    Avoid minimising or overstating the situation. Be factual, but show compassion and understanding.
4. Provide clear information :
    Make sure the patient understands the situation. It may be helpful to provide written information or additional resources.
5. Encourage questions :
    Let the patient express their concerns and ask questions to clarify their understanding.
6. Recognising unfulfilled expectations :
    Talk openly about the hopes or expectations the patient initially had, and discuss the reasons why these results were not achieved.
7. Propose solutions or alternatives :
    If possible, offer options for the future, whether in terms of other interventions, complementary treatments or psychological support.
8. Allowing time :
    Let the patient process the news. It may be useful to schedule another appointment to discuss the matter in more detail or to answer any further questions.

Communicating difficult news requires sensitivity, patience and honesty. Maxillo-facial surgery professionals, faced with the aesthetic and functional hopes of patients, must be particularly attentive to this dimension of the care-giver-patient relationship. By adopting a patient-centred approach and using effective communication techniques, it is possible to navigate these delicate situations with dignity and compassion.

Supporting families and loved ones in times of stress

In the world of maxillofacial surgery, the focus is often on the patient, but behind every patient is a family or loved ones who are also going through this ordeal. Surgery of any kind inevitably generates stress and anxiety, not only for the patient but also for those around them. These emotions can be exacerbated by uncertainty, fear of the unknown, and the aesthetic and functional implications of maxillofacial procedures.

As a healthcare professional, it is essential to understand the crucial role that family and friends play in a patient's recovery and well-being. They are often the main source of support, offering comfort, encouragement and practical assistance.
Recognising their needs, concerns and feelings is an essential step in ensuring holistic care. This means offering clear, up-to-date information about the procedure, recovery and possible complications, so that relatives can feel informed and involved.

But beyond providing information, it is just as important to provide emotional support. Clinics and hospitals could consider organising group sessions for families, offering a space to share experiences, ask questions and receive mutual support. Relatives, like patients, can benefit from counselling or therapy to help them manage the stress and anxiety associated with surgery.

It is also essential to encourage open communication. Invite families to express their concerns, ask questions and share their feelings. When they feel heard and understood, they are better equipped to support their loved one during the post-operative period.

The key is collaboration. By working in partnership with relatives, actively involving them in the care process and recognising their essential role, we can provide a reassuring and healing environment for the patient.

In conclusion, if the patient is at the heart of the maxillofacial surgery care process, those close to him or her are its foundation. By offering support, information and understanding to these individuals, we not only help the patient in his or her recovery, but we also strengthen the fabric of support around the patient, creating a stronger and more effective dynamic of care.

Chapter 13:
EMERGENCY MANAGEMENT
IN MAXILLO-FACIAL SURGERY

Emergency response protocols

In the field of maxillofacial surgery, emergency situations can arise suddenly, requiring rapid, coordinated and precise action to ensure the patient's safety and well-being. These situations can range from facial trauma to post-operative haemorrhage and severe infections. So having well-established emergency response protocols is vital.

1. Initial assessment and triage :
On arrival in an emergency, a rapid but thorough assessment is crucial. The patient's vital signs, such as breathing, pulse and blood pressure, must be checked immediately. Similarly, assessment of consciousness, respiratory capacity and haemodynamic stability is essential.

2. Airway management :
Protecting and maintaining the airway is the top priority. Maxillofacial trauma can lead to obstruction, and intubation or even tracheostomy may be necessary in an **emergency.**

3. Bleeding control :
Facial injuries can bleed profusely due to the rich vascularity of the area. Direct compression is the first step, followed by an assessment to determine whether surgery is necessary to stop the bleeding.

4. Assessment of lesions :
Once the patient's situation has stabilised, a full assessment of the injuries must be carried out. This includes a physical examination, X-rays and other imaging techniques to determine the extent of the injuries.

5. Management of fractures :

Fractures need to be stabilised to prevent further injury and to prepare for possible surgery. This may involve the use of splints or other devices.

6. Treatment of infections :

Serious infections require rapid intervention, including the administration of antibiotics. If a source of infection is identified, such as an abscess, it may require incision and drainage.

7. Communication and coordination :

Clear communication between all members of the medical team is essential. Surgeons, anaesthetists, nurses and radiologists must work in harmony to ensure optimal care.

8. Monitoring and reassessment :

After the initial treatment, the patient must be regularly monitored and reassessed to ensure that his or her condition remains stable and that other complications do not develop.

Maxillofacial surgery, because of its complexity and vital importance, requires impeccable preparation and responsiveness in the event of an emergency. Emergency response protocols are designed to guide healthcare professionals through the crucial steps to save lives, preserve function and minimise long-term sequelae. These protocols, combined with regular training and practical exercises, ensure that the team is always ready to act in any emergency situation.

Working together
with the emergency services

Inter-departmental collaboration, particularly between maxillofacial surgery departments and emergency services, is fundamental to ensuring optimal patient care. Trauma to the face, whether accidental or pathological, is frequently first treated by emergency services before being referred to maxillo-facial surgery specialists. The smoothness of this transition, based on close collaboration, is vital to the patient's safety and well-being.

1. Common protocols and cross-training :
It is essential that emergency department and maxillofacial surgery teams share common protocols for the initial management of facial injuries. This may include cross-training where maxillofacial surgeons attend emergency department training sessions and vice versa.

2. Effective communication :
The rapid exchange of accurate clinical information is crucial. The use of integrated electronic medical record systems, direct communication channels and telemedicine tools can facilitate this exchange.

3. Transfers and guidelines :
Clearly established procedures for transferring patients between departments can speed up management, minimise duplication of tests and reduce waiting time for the patient.

4. Regular interdisciplinary meetings :
Organising regular meetings between the two departments allows cases to be discussed, experiences to be shared and procedures to be constantly improved. These meetings also foster a better mutual understanding of roles and responsibilities.

5. Simulation scenarios and practical exercises :
Setting up simulations of maxillofacial emergencies can help prepare teams to work together in a coordinated way in real-life situations. These simulations can cover scenarios such as serious facial trauma, major haemorrhage or airway obstruction.

6. Continuity of care :
Post-operation follow-up is essential. The emergency services must be kept informed of the results of the operation and the post-operative follow-up so that they have an overview of the patient's care.

7. Patient and family education :
The two services should work together to provide patients and their families with clear and consistent information about the nature of the injury, the planned interventions and post-operative care.

Collaboration between maxillofacial surgery departments and emergency services is a necessary alliance to ensure fast, efficient and high-quality care for patients. This synergy requires open communication, ongoing training and a mutual understanding of the roles and responsibilities of each department. Ultimately, it is the patient who benefits most from this close collaboration, through coordinated and optimised care.

Post-emergency psychological support for patients and staff

When it comes to facial trauma and complex maxillofacial surgery procedures, the psychological impact is often as profound as the physical implications. The facial region plays a central role in personal identity, non-verbal communication and social interaction. Trauma or interventions in this area can have major emotional repercussions, both for the patient and for the medical team involved. Psychological support after an emergency is therefore essential for full recovery.

1. For patients :

Early identification: All patients undergoing maxillofacial surgery should be assessed for psychological distress. This enables early signs of anxiety, depression or other disorders to be identified and appropriate support to be provided.

Counselling: Counselling can help patients understand and process their emotions. Regular follow-up with a trained professional can address issues such as self-perception, physical concerns and social reintegration.

Support groups: Meeting others who have been through similar experiences can provide valuable insight and a sense of camaraderie.

Education: Understanding the nature of the injury, the healing process and post-operative expectations can reduce anxiety.

2. For the medical team :

Post-emergency debriefing: After a particularly difficult or traumatic intervention, it is essential to bring the team together to discuss the experience. This is an opportunity to express emotions, clarify events and get support from colleagues.

Training in empathic communication: Learning to communicate with compassion and empathy can help the medical team to interact better with traumatised patients and their families.

Access to professional support: Psychologists or social workers should be available to the team, either for individual sessions or support groups.

Stress management: Relaxation techniques, meditation and other stress management methods can be beneficial for the team, especially after long and complex operations.

Post-emergency psychological support is a crucial component of care in maxillofacial surgery. While injuries or deformities can heal over time, emotional scars require dedicated care and attention. By taking into account the emotional well-being of the patient and the team, the healing process can be more complete, faster and more holistic.

Chapter 14:
PREVENTION AND EDUCATION FOR PATIENTS

Prevention and education are the cornerstones of modern medicine. In maxillofacial surgery, they are of paramount importance, not only to avoid possible interventions, but also to prepare and inform patients before and after surgery. Together, these two elements contribute to better overall management, reducing risks and improving results.

In terms of prevention, it is essential to make patients aware of the risk situations that could lead to maxillofacial trauma. This may involve advice on road safety, such as wearing seatbelts, using helmets on two-wheelers, or the importance of avoiding risky behaviour, such as driving under the influence. And when it comes to contact sports, the use of protective equipment such as mouthguards can prevent many injuries.

Education takes place throughout the patient's medical career. Before an operation, it is vital to inform the patient of the exact nature of the procedure, its benefits and risks, and the post-operative care required. Proper understanding enables patients to play an active part in their recovery, thereby reducing the risk of complications.

After the operation, education continues to play a key role. Patients need to be fully informed about care at home, how to recognise signs of infection or other complications, and what steps to take to ensure optimal recovery. Education also includes information on appropriate nutrition, pain management, and any complementary therapies that may help recovery.

Prevention and education, when properly integrated into the care pathway, form a strong alliance. They not only help to minimise interventions, but also ensure that each intervention is as safe and effective as possible. Patients are then better prepared, more autonomous and often more satisfied with the process and the results obtained. It is therefore essential for all maxillofacial surgery professionals to consider these two aspects as an integral part of their mission, for the well-being and optimum health of their patients.

Prevention of facial trauma

The face, the seat of our identity and expression, is also an anatomically complex region that is particularly vulnerable to injury. Facial trauma can be devastating both functionally and aesthetically. It is therefore essential to implement preventive strategies to reduce the incidence and severity of these injuries.

1. Raising awareness of road safety :
A large proportion of facial injuries are caused by road accidents. Promoting the use of seatbelts and helmets for cyclists and motorcyclists is crucial. It is also vital to instil the importance of not driving under the influence of alcohol, drugs or when tired.

2. Sports and leisure activities :
Contact sports such as rugby, hockey or boxing present an increased risk of facial injuries. The use of mouthguards, helmets with face protection grids and other specific equipment can prevent a large proportion of these injuries. Coaches and sports institutions are responsible for encouraging and implementing these safety measures.

3. Work environment :
In certain professions, such as construction or industry, the risk of facial injuries is higher. Wearing safety glasses,

helmets and masks can greatly reduce these risks. Regular training on safety and prevention in the workplace is essential.

4. Home prevention :
Many accidents happen in the home. Whether it's falls, accidents with tools or incidents in the kitchen, being aware of the dangers in the home and taking simple precautions can prevent many injuries.

5. Community awareness :
Education and awareness-raising play a major role in prevention. Local campaigns, workshops and school programmes dedicated to trauma prevention can have a significant impact.

6. Research and innovation:
Ongoing safety research, such as the development of better-performing helmets or safer vehicles, also helps to reduce facial injuries.

Preventing facial trauma is not just a matter of common sense or individual prudence. It requires a multi-dimensional approach, involving education, awareness, research and the implementation of strict safety regulations. By working together, we can significantly reduce injuries and their consequences, preserving everyone's health and quality of life.

Education on post-operative care

When a patient undergoes maxillofacial surgery, the post-operative phase is just as crucial as the operation itself in ensuring optimal recovery. Informing the patient and, where appropriate, his or her next of kin, is essential to ensure that appropriate post-operative care is followed and that the risk of complications is minimised.

1. Pain management :
One of the main concerns after surgery is pain. It is crucial to inform the patient about the analgesics prescribed, their dosage, any side effects and how long they should be taken. It is also important to report any excessive or prolonged pain.

2. Care of the wound :
The operated area requires specific care to prevent infection and promote healing. Clear instructions on how to clean the wound, how often to dress it and what signs of infection to look out for (redness, heat, purulent discharge) are essential.

3. Diet and oral hygiene :
Depending on the nature of the operation, dietary restrictions may be necessary. Recommendations on the type of food, its consistency (liquid, soft), as well as advice on post-operative oral hygiene, such as the use of antiseptic mouthwashes or the appropriate brushing technique, can be given.

4. Physical activity and rest :
The appropriate level of post-operative activity should be clearly defined to avoid strain or pressure on the operated area. Guidelines on how long to rest, what activities to avoid, and when to resume exercise or return to work are crucial.

5. Medical follow-up and check-ups:
Patients must be informed of any necessary post-operative appointments, examinations, or rehabilitation sessions, to ensure that recovery proceeds as planned.

6. Warning signs :
It is imperative to make patients aware of signs indicating possible complications, such as excessive bleeding, sudden swelling, intense pain, numbness, or breathing problems.

7. Psychological aspects :
Maxillofacial surgery can have aesthetic implications, and it is essential to address the issue of self-perception after

surgery, encouraging the patient to discuss their feelings and, if necessary, consider psychological support.

Post-operative education is an essential part of surgical management. Clear communication, appropriate educational resources and regular follow-up ensure that patients are well equipped to navigate the post-operative period, ensuring the best possible outcomes for their health and well-being.

Raising awareness of the risks associated with tobacco, alcohol and other factors

Maxillofacial surgery is a speciality that focuses on a particularly sensitive area of the human body: the face and mouth. External factors such as smoking, excessive alcohol consumption and other substances can have a direct impact on oral and facial health, as well as on the success of surgical procedures.

1. Tobacco: a silent threat
Smoking is one of the greatest enemies of oral health. Not only is it a major cause of oral cancer, but it also hinders the body's ability to heal after surgery.

Effects on oral health: As well as cancer, smoking is linked to periodontitis, tooth discolouration and bad breath.

Post-operative risks: Smokers have an increased risk of complications after surgery, including infections, scarring problems and less aesthetically pleasing results.

2. Alcohol: not just a liver issue
Excessive alcohol consumption not only harms the liver; it

can also have disastrous consequences for oral and maxillofacial health.

> **Effects on oral health**: Alcohol dries out the mouth, encouraging bacterial growth. It is also a risk factor for oral cancer, especially when combined with smoking.

> **Surgical consequences**: Alcohol consumption can increase bleeding during and after surgery. It can also interact with prescribed medication and affect healing.

3. Other factors to consider

As well as tobacco and alcohol, other substances and behaviours can damage maxillofacial health. Drugs, poor diet and neglected oral hygiene can aggravate pre-existing conditions or create new ones.

4. Prevention as the first line of defence

Educating patients about the dangers of tobacco, alcohol and other risk factors is essential. By highlighting the risks, offering resources for quitting smoking or reducing alcohol consumption, and encouraging a healthy lifestyle, nurses play a crucial role in preventing maxillofacial health problems.

Maxillo-facial surgery does not stop in the operating theatre. Prevention, education and awareness of modifiable risks are an essential part of overall patient care. By adopting a proactive approach, it is possible to reduce the number of cases requiring intervention and considerably improve patients' quality of life.

Chapter 15:
INFECTIONS AND COMPLICATIONS POST-OPERATIVE

Recognise early signs of infection

The human body has an incredible capacity to heal itself, but in certain circumstances an injury, surgery or illness can lead to infection. In maxillofacial surgery, as in other medical specialities, prompt management of infections is vital to prevent more serious complications. To do this, it is essential to recognise the early signs of infection.

1. Redness and local heat
One of the first signs of infection is redness of the skin around the affected area. This is often associated with a sensation of warmth to the touch. These symptoms are due to an increase in blood flow to the infected area, the body's natural defence mechanism.

2. Swelling or oedema
Swelling is often a sign of an accumulation of fluid, immune cells and bacteria in the affected area. In maxillofacial surgery, this can be seen around the mouth, neck or face.

3. Pain or increased sensitivity
Pain is the body's reaction to an aggressor. An infected area is often painful to the touch or spontaneously. Pain may increase progressively as the infection develops.

4. Pus or discharge
The presence of pus is a clear sign of infection. It is a thick liquid, often white, yellow or green in colour, containing immune cells, dead bacteria and living or dead tissue.

5. Fever and chills
A fever is the body's response to an infection. It helps the body fight bacteria or viruses by creating an environment

less conducive to their multiplication. Chills are often a sign of a rapid rise in body temperature.

6. Fatigue or general malaise

When the body is fighting an infection, it's common to feel tired or generally unwell.

7. Bad breath or unpleasant taste in the mouth

In the event of an oral infection, the multiplication of bacteria can lead to bad breath or an unpleasant taste.

Recognising the early signs of infection is crucial to rapid and effective treatment. In maxillofacial surgery, where the face and mouth are at stake, this is particularly important. It is therefore essential for patients, nurses and doctors to be alert to these symptoms, take them seriously and treat them quickly to avoid complications.

Infection management protocols

Maxillofacial surgery, which focuses on the essential structures of the face and mouth, requires particular attention to infection prevention and management. An infection in this area can quickly become serious due to the proximity of the respiratory tract, nerves and major blood vessels. Here is an overview of the infection management protocols specific to this speciality.

1. Pre-operative prevention

- **Antibiotic prophylaxis**: Administration of antibiotics prior to surgery to reduce the risk of post-operative infection, particularly for major surgery or immunocompromised patients.
- **Skin preparation**: rigorous cleaning and antisepsis of the operating area with appropriate antiseptic solutions.

2. Early identification

Regular monitoring: Daily examination for signs of infection such as redness, warmth, swelling, pain or pus discharge.

Laboratory tests: Prescription of blood tests to detect an increase in white blood cells or other signs of infection.

3. Active management

Culture and antibiotic susceptibility test: Collection of any discharge or pus to identify the pathogen and determine the most appropriate antibiotic.

Targeted antibiotic therapy: Initiation or adjustment of antibiotics according to the results of the antibiogram to ensure effective action against the bacteria in question.

Surgical drainage: In some cases, evacuation of the pus or infected fluid is necessary to reduce the bacterial load and improve the effectiveness of antibiotics.

4. Local care

Regular cleaning: Use mild cleaning solutions to keep the area clean.

Antimicrobial dressings: Use of dressings impregnated with antimicrobial agents to reduce bacterial proliferation.

Protection: Ensure that the infected area is well protected to prevent further contamination.

5. Post-operative follow-up

Patient education: Inform the patient about the signs of infection and the importance of regular post-operative monitoring.

Follow-up visits: Examine the patient regularly to ensure resolution of the infection and to anticipate any signs of complications.

6. Reassessment

If, despite all treatment, the infection persists or worsens, a full reassessment is necessary. This may involve further surgery, changes in antibiotics or further investigations to identify a possible underlying cause.

Infection management in maxillofacial surgery is essential to ensure patient safety and well-being. The combination of rigorous prevention, early identification and active infection management, reinforced by patient education and close post-operative follow-up, is the key to minimising risk and ensuring the best possible outcomes.

Specific complications maxillo-facial surgery

Maxillofacial surgery, which focuses on the face, jaw and mouth, presents distinct challenges and is subject to specific complications. Here's a look at these complications, which are essential for any professional working in this field to be aware of.

1. Haemorrhage and haematoma
    - **Origin**: The face and neck are full of blood vessels, some of them of major importance. Injury to these vessels can lead to significant bleeding.
    - **Management**: Local compression, surgical revision for ligation, and sometimes blood transfusion.
2. Infection
    - **Origin**: Despite asepsis protocols, the risk of infection remains, particularly due to the proximity of the oral cavity, which is naturally colonised by bacteria.
    - **Management**: Antibiotic therapy, surgical drainage and local care.
3. Tissue necrosis
    - **Origin**: Poor post-operative vascularisation can compromise tissue survival.
    - **Management**: Reintervention, local care and, in some cases, recourse to reconstruction procedures.

4. Nerve damage

   Origin: Facial nerves, particularly the facial nerve, can be damaged during surgery, resulting in paralysis or paresthesia.

   Management: Observation, physiotherapy and sometimes reconstructive surgery.

5. Aesthetic problems and asymmetries

   Origin: Despite the precautions taken, surgery can result in unsightly scars or asymmetries.

   Management: Surgical revisions, laser treatments, filling therapies and psychological support.

6. Ocular complications

   Origin: Surgery close to the orbit can lead to complications such as ectropion, entropion, or even direct ocular lesions.

   Management: Medical treatment, protective eyewear, eye surgery.

7. Breathing difficulties

   Origin: Operations on the jaw or near the airways can lead to oedema or obstruction.

   Management: Monitoring in intensive care unit, intubation or tracheostomy in an emergency.

8. Malocclusion

   Origin: Teeth alignment problems can occur after jaw surgery.

   Management: Orthodontics, dental adjustments or corrective surgery.

9. Orosinus or oroantral fistulas

   Origin: These are abnormal communications between the mouth and the sinuses or nasal cavity.

   Management: Surgical closure, antibiotics and appropriate dental care.

Every maxillofacial surgery is unique, and the risk of complications varies depending on the procedure, the patient and the circumstances. In-depth knowledge of potential complications, combined with impeccable surgical technique, rigorous preparation and careful post-operative monitoring, is essential to optimise results and patient safety.

Chapter 16:
THE CHALLENGES OF REHABILITATION AND PHYSIOTHERAPY

Assessment and implementation rehabilitation plans

The art of maxillofacial surgery does not stop in the operating theatre. Rehabilitation, the crucial stage after any surgical intervention, requires rigorous assessment and the implementation of tailored plans to ensure optimal healing and a gradual return to normality for the patient.

1. Initial post-operative assessment

   Clinical examination: A thorough assessment of the surgical site is essential to detect any early signs of complications.

   Pain assessment: Pain management is a fundamental aspect of convalescence. Regular assessment, using pain scales, enables analgesic treatment to be adjusted.

   Functional assessment: Assessing masticatory, phonatory and respiratory functions is essential to understanding the patient's immediate rehabilitation needs.

2. Drawing up a rehabilitation plan

   Functional rehabilitation: Engaging the patient in targeted exercises to restore function, whether in mandibular movements, speech or other orofacial functions.

   Wound care: Advice on cleaning, dressing and monitoring wounds can help prevent complications and promote rapid healing.

   Adapted nutrition: Offer an adapted diet, often soft or liquid, which evolves as recovery progresses.

3. Monitoring and reassessments
- **Regular consultations**: Post-operative visits are used to assess the progress of recovery, detect any complications and adjust the rehabilitation plan.
- **Checking for late complications**: Problems such as joint ankylosis, masticatory dysfunctions or aesthetic problems may appear weeks or even months after the operation.

4. Psychological support
- **Emotional repercussions**: Maxillo-facial surgery can have a considerable impact on body image. It is vital to offer psychological support to help patients accept and adapt to these changes.
- **Support groups**: Referring patients to support groups or community resources can provide them with perspective and coping strategies.

5. Interdisciplinary collaboration
- **Teamwork**: Speech therapists, physiotherapists, dieticians, psychologists and other professionals can play an essential role in the rehabilitation plan.
- **Sharing information**: Ensuring fluid communication between all those involved in the care of a patient enables holistic care to be provided.

Rehabilitation after maxillofacial surgery is a path strewn with obstacles and challenges. However, with a thorough assessment, a tailored care plan, a dedicated team and patient support, the results can be not only functional, but also life-changing, restoring patients' confidence in themselves and their future.

Specialised physiotherapy techniques

Maxillofacial surgery, which focuses on the structure and function of the face, jaw and neck, can leave patients with functional limitations, pain or cosmetic problems after the operation. Physiotherapy plays an essential role in post-operative rehabilitation, aiming to restore function, reduce pain and optimise aesthetic appearance.

1. Manual therapy

Joint mobilisation: These techniques aim to restore normal mobility to the temporomandibular and cervical joints.

Myofascial massage: By focusing on releasing tension and adhesions in the fascia, this technique can improve tissue mobility and reduce pain.

2. Therapeutic exercises

Masticatory rehabilitation: Specific exercises to strengthen and improve coordination of the masticatory muscles.

Swallowing rehabilitation: For patients with post-operative swallowing difficulties.

Posture and cervical strengthening exercises: Encouraging optimal posture to reduce unnecessary tension in the operated area.

3. Neuromuscular techniques

Electrotherapy: Use of electrical currents to stimulate muscle contraction, reduce pain and promote healing.

Biofeedback: A technique in which patients receive real-time information about their muscular function, helping them to improve their control.

4. Manual lymph drainage

Reducing oedema: Using gentle, rhythmic movements, the therapist encourages excess fluid to drain from the operated area, thereby reducing swelling.

5. Thermal techniques

Cryotherapy: Applying ice can help reduce inflammation and post-operative pain.

Thermotherapy: Heat can relax tense muscles and improve blood circulation in the operated area.

6. Patient education

- **Self-management strategies**: Educating patients about techniques they can use at home to manage their pain, mobility or other symptoms.
- **Preventive advice**: Advice on posture, sleeping habits and stretching techniques to avoid possible recurrences or complications.

Specialist physiotherapy for patients who have undergone maxillofacial surgery is a dynamic collaboration between therapist and patient. By combining clinically proven techniques with personalised education, it provides patients with the tools and skills they need to make a full recovery and return to a normal life.

Working with speech therapists and other therapists

In the vast world of medicine, maxillo-facial surgery occupies a special place, touching on both aesthetics and the essential function of the face. The complexity of this speciality requires seamless inter-professional collaboration. Speech therapists, who specialise in speech and swallowing disorders, are among the key players in this multidisciplinary team.

A patient who has undergone maxillofacial surgery may have after-effects that affect his or her ability to speak or swallow. The speech therapist's intervention is therefore essential. Using specific techniques, the speech therapist will work to restore and optimise these essential functions, with a direct impact on the patient's quality of life. It is not uncommon for patients to experience discomfort, a change in voice or difficulty in articulating following an operation. Thanks to the expertise of the speech therapist, a personalised programme is put in place, aimed at restoring fluent speech and easy swallowing.

But collaboration doesn't stop there. Post-operative care in maxillofacial surgery often involves a multitude of health professionals. Physiotherapists, for example, play a crucial role in functional rehabilitation, working on neck and jaw mobility, while nutritionists ensure that the patient's diet is adapted to his or her chewing and swallowing abilities. Psychologists may also be involved, offering emotional support in the face of the challenges and changes the patient may encounter.

This synergy between healthcare professionals guarantees comprehensive patient care, where every detail and every possible complication is anticipated and dealt with. The role of the nurse in this collaboration is central. As the linchpin of care coordination, they are in direct contact with each of these specialists, ensuring fluid, effective communication that is essential to the success of the care pathway.

So far from being an isolated procedure, maxillofacial surgery is part of a holistic approach, in which every professional - from speech therapist to physiotherapist, from nutritionist to psychologist - makes their own contribution, working hand in hand to offer patients the best possible quality of life.

Chapter 17:
PAIN MANAGEMENT

Pain assessment

Pain is an unpleasant sensory and emotional experience associated with actual or potential tissue damage. In maxillofacial surgery, accurate assessment of pain is fundamental, not only to ensure patient comfort, but also to prevent possible post-operative complications. This assessment must be multidimensional, taking into account the intensity, location, nature and duration of the pain, as well as its impact on the patient's quality of life.

Pain intensity is often measured using verbal, numerical or visual scales, giving patients the opportunity to quantify how they feel. A simple "From 0 to 10, how would you rate your pain?" can provide valuable information to the medical team. However, these scales have their limitations, particularly in the case of children, the elderly or people with communication difficulties.

The location of the pain makes it possible to pinpoint the origin of the problem. In maxillofacial surgery, pain can originate in the jaw, teeth, gums, face or surrounding soft tissue. Precise pain mapping facilitates diagnosis and appropriate treatment.

The nature of the pain, whether it is stabbing, throbbing, dull or acute, can point to different aetiologies. Post-operative pain is often acute and diminishes over time, while chronic pain may be the sign of a complication or underlying pathology.

The assessment must also take into account the impact of the pain on the patient's daily life: disturbed sleep, difficulty eating or speaking, altered mood, etc. These factors, although subjective, are essential for adapting treatment and providing comprehensive care.

Finally, it is crucial to assess pain regularly, especially after surgery. The evolution of pain, its intensification or attenuation, can provide indications of the healing process or the appearance of complications.

The nurse plays a central role here, often being the patient's first point of contact. By being close at hand and available, they are able to gather precise information, reassure the patient and adjust the analgesic treatment if necessary. Working closely with the medical team, nurses play an active role in pain assessment and management, ensuring that maxillofacial surgery patients receive optimum care.

Specific analgesic protocols

Pain management is crucial in maxillofacial surgery, not only to ensure patient comfort but also to promote rapid and effective recovery. Analgesic protocols specific to this speciality take into account the nature and extent of the operation, as well as the patient's individual needs.

Initial pain assessment :
    Before any analgesic   is administered, a full pain assessment is essential. This enables the intensity, location and nature of the pain to be determined. Assessment scales, such as the Visual Analogue Scale (VAS), are invaluable tools in this respect.

Multimodal analgesia :

The multimodal approach involves combining different analgesic drugs to optimise pain relief while minimising side effects. For example, a non-steroidal anti-inflammatory drug (NSAID) may be combined with paracetamol, or even opioids for more intense pain.

Nerve blocks :

For some operations, a nerve block can be used to anaesthetise a specific area of the face. This not only reduces post-operative pain but also reduces the need for other analgesics.

Opioids :

In the event of severe pain, opioids such as morphine, fentanyl or oxycodone may be prescribed. However, because of their addictive potential and side effects (nausea, constipation, drowsiness, etc.), their use must be carefully monitored.

Taking drug interactions into account :

Some patients may be taking medication for other conditions. It is therefore essential to assess possible interactions between analgesics and these drugs.

Managing side effects :

The administration of analgesics can lead to side effects. Regular monitoring enables these to be detected early and treatment adjusted accordingly.

Regular reassessment :

Pain must be assessed regularly, and the analgesic protocol adapted according to the evolution of the pain and the patient's needs.

Patient education :

It is crucial to inform patients about pain management at home, including the importance of adhering to prescribed doses and reporting any adverse effects.

Maxillo-facial surgery nurses play a vital role in implementing and monitoring analgesic protocols. By listening to patients and applying their expertise, they ensure their well-being, guaranteeing optimal, personalised pain management.

Non-medicinal techniques pain management

Pain, as a complex phenomenon, can be influenced by physiological, psychological and social factors. In maxillofacial surgery, although drugs are the first line of treatment for post-operative pain, it is increasingly common to complement this drug-based approach with non-drug techniques. These techniques have the advantage of reducing the need for analgesics, minimising side effects and offering patients comprehensive pain management.

Manual therapies :
   Massage: This technique helps to relax muscles, improve blood circulation and encourage the secretion of endorphins, the body's natural painkillers.
   Physiotherapy: Specific movements and mobilisation exercises can help relieve pain and prevent post-operative stiffness.
Cognitive-behavioural therapies :
   Relaxation and deep breathing: These techniques help to reduce stress, anxiety and muscular tension, all of which can amplify the perception of pain.
   Medical   hypnosis: This changes the perception of pain and makes it easier to relax.
Distraction techniques :

- **Music therapy**: Listening to music or taking part in music therapy sessions can reduce pain and anxiety.
- **Virtual reality**: Immersion in a virtual environment can distract patients from their pain.

Transcutaneous electrical stimulation (TENS) :

This technique uses electrical impulses to stimulate the nerves, blocking the transmission of pain.

Thermotherapy and cryotherapy :

- Applying heat can relax muscles and improve circulation, helping to relieve pain.
- Applying cold can reduce inflammation and numb the painful area.

Acupuncture and acupressure :

These traditional Chinese techniques can help relieve pain by stimulating specific points on the body.

Biofeedback :

This technique teaches patients to control certain physiological functions (such as heart rate) to help them manage their pain.

Aromatherapy :

Using specific essential oils can help reduce pain and anxiety.

By incorporating these non-medicinal techniques into their care protocols, maxillo-facial surgery nurses can offer patients holistic pain management. However, it is essential to tailor this management to the patient's needs and preferences, and to regularly assess its effectiveness.

Chapter 18:
PAEDIATRIC MAXILLO-FACIAL SURGERY

Anatomical differences
and physiology in children

The management of children in maxillofacial surgery presents particular challenges due to the anatomical and physiological differences that distinguish them from adults. A thorough understanding of these variations is crucial to providing appropriate and safe care for the youngest patients.

Skull and face :

Fontanelles: Babies are born with soft areas on their skull, called fontanelles, which gradually close as they grow.

Proportions : A child's head is proportionally larger than an adult's in relation to the rest of the body.

Sinuses: The frontal sinuses only start to develop after the age of two and are not fully formed until adolescence.

Dentition :

Children have a first set of teeth, the milk teeth, which gradually fall out to make way for the permanent dentition.

Tooth eruption can vary considerably from one child to another.

Respiratory tract :

Size: Children's airways are narrower, making them more susceptible to obstructions.

Epiglottis: Larger and less flexible in children, increasing the risk of obstruction.

- **Tongue**: Proportionately larger than the mouth.
- Circulatory system :
    - **Heart rate**: Children have a higher heart rate and a higher basal metabolic rate.
    - **Blood volume**: Even minimal blood loss during an operation can have more serious consequences for a child because of its low total blood volume.
- Bone and soft tissue :
    - **Bone growth**: Growth plates (epiphyses) are areas of active cartilage tissue where bone growth occurs and which are sensitive to injury.
    - **Tissue elasticity**: Children's skin and tissue are more elastic, which can affect suturing techniques.
- Physiological response :
    - Children may have a different physiological response to medicines, requiring dosages to be adjusted.
    - Their ability to regulate temperature is less developed, making them more vulnerable to temperature variations.
- Cognitive and emotional development :
    - Children don't always understand what's happening to them, which can lead to anxiety.
    - They may find it difficult to communicate their pain or discomfort.

These differences, among others, require specialised training for professionals working in paediatric maxillofacial surgery. The approach to care must be adapted not only to the child's anatomical and physiological needs, but also to his or her psychological and emotional needs.

Specific challenges paediatric care

Maxillofacial surgery in children is a delicate area, requiring particular expertise. In addition to anatomical and physiological differences, there are many other challenges unique to paediatric care in this area.

- Limited understanding :
  - Children may not understand the need for surgery, making pre-operative preparation more difficult. Explaining in a way that is adapted to their age and level of understanding is crucial.
- Managing anxiety :
  - The operating theatre can be an intimidating environment for a child. Fear of the unknown, separation from parents and exposure to surgical instruments can cause great anxiety.
- Pharmacological considerations :
  - Children react differently to medicines than adults. The dosage, administration and monitoring of side effects require special attention.
- Communication :
  - Depending on their age, children may not be able to express their pain or discomfort clearly, requiring appropriate assessment methods.
- Informed consent :
  - Although older children can contribute to decision-making, it is usually up to the parents or guardians to give their consent. This can sometimes lead to complex situations where the child's wishes differ from those of the parents.

Long-term implications :
> Surgical interventions can have implications for a child's future   growth and development. It is essential to consider these impacts when planning surgery.

Psychosocial aspects :
> Scars or changes in appearance can have psychosocial implications for the child, particularly in terms of self-esteem and social integration.

Family and friends :
> Parents or relatives are deeply involved in the child's care and recovery. Their support, understanding and cooperation are essential, but they may also need emotional support.

Multidisciplinary coordination :
> Treating children in maxillofacial surgery often requires collaboration with other specialities such as paediatrics, orthodontics, speech therapy and psychology, among others.

Ethical aspects :
Ethical dilemmas may arise, for example, concerning cosmetic procedures on children or major procedures with significant risks.

Paediatric maxillofacial surgery requires greater expertise, sensitivity and adaptability. Caregivers must not only focus on the technical aspects of surgery, but also consider the emotional and psychological needs of the child and his or her family.

Collaboration
with paediatric services

Collaboration between maxillo-facial surgery and paediatric services is essential for optimal care of young patients. This interaction is fundamental, as children have anatomical, physiological, psychological and developmental particularities that require a specific approach.

Pre-operative assessment :
The collaboration often begins with a joint pre-operative assessment. The paediatrician assesses the child's general condition, medical history and any concomitant conditions that may affect the operation.

Psychological preparation :
Paediatric psychologists can help prepare the child and family for the procedure. They provide strategies for managing anxiety and helping the child to understand what is going to happen.

Adapting protocols :
Anaesthetic and surgical protocols are adapted to children's physiology. Collaboration ensures that these protocols comply with best paediatric practice.

Communication :
Clear communication is crucial. The surgical and paediatric teams must share relevant information about the child's condition, the planned procedures and the expected results.

Post-operative follow-up :
After the operation, follow-up is often carried out jointly. The maxillo-facial surgeon will be interested in the outcome of the operation,

while the paediatrician will monitor the child for any general complications.

Rehabilitation and therapy :

In some cases, the child may need rehabilitation, for example with a speech therapist for speech or a physiotherapist for muscle function. Close collaboration ensures a coordinated treatment plan.

Multidisciplinary meetings:

Regular meetings between the different teams enable complex cases to be examined, the best treatment options to be discussed and care to be coordinated.

Training and education :

Ongoing training is essential. Paediatric teams can offer training on the particularities of paediatric care, while the maxillofacial surgery team can share knowledge on specific surgical techniques.

Joint research :

The two departments can collaborate on studies and research to improve techniques, results and patient care.

Collaboration between maxillo-facial surgery and paediatric services is essential to ensure holistic care for children. This synergy not only improves clinical outcomes but also the overall experience for the child and their family.

Chapter 19:
CRISIS MANAGEMENT
AND EXTREME CASES

Responding to disasters and emergencies

Faced with a disaster or emergency situation, the need to intervene quickly and effectively is imperative. In the field of maxillofacial surgery, these interventions can involve major facial trauma resulting from accidents, natural disasters or armed conflicts. Dealing with such operations requires specific preparation, interdisciplinary coordination and rapid action protocols.

Preparation and training :
> Emergency training is crucial. Professionals must be trained in emergency procedures, the specific protocols to be followed and the use of specialised equipment.

Victim triage :
> In disaster situations, rapid triage is essential to identify patients who require immediate intervention, those who can wait, and those for whom care would be futile. Maxillofacial injuries can compromise the airway, requiring rapid intervention.

Patient stabilisation :
> The priority is to stabilise patients, ensuring a free airway, controlling bleeding and treating associated trauma.

Emergency surgery :
> Complex fractures, deep lesions and trauma associated with other injuries may require immediate surgery. Interventions can range

from the placement of drains to reconstructive surgery.

- Logistics and equipment :
  - Having the right surgical equipment and trained staff is crucial. In disaster zones, this may involve mobile surgical units, specific emergency kits and effective communication systems.
- Interdisciplinary coordination :
  - Maxillo-facial surgery never takes place in a vacuum. It requires close collaboration with other specialities such as anaesthesia, traumatology, neurosurgery and even psychology.
- Post-operative care and rehabilitation :
  - After initial operations, patients require appropriate post-operative care to prevent infection, manage pain and initiate rehabilitation. In disaster situations, this can be a challenge due to limited resources.
- Psychosocial support :
  - Physical trauma is often accompanied by psychological trauma. Mental health professionals can intervene to help patients deal with shock, post-traumatic stress and rehabilitation.
- Feedback and continuous improvement:
  - After each intervention in a disaster situation, it is vital to debrief, gather feedback and adjust protocols accordingly to improve future responses.

The ability to respond effectively in a disaster situation is the result of careful preparation, effective coordination and ongoing training. The challenges are many, but with a structured and collaborative approach, maxillofacial surgery teams can provide vital care in times of crisis.

Management of extreme cases: major burns, war trauma

Extreme cases in maxillofacial surgery, such as severe burns or war-related trauma, present unique challenges. These situations require not only advanced surgical skills, but also a holistic approach to managing patients' medical, psychological and social needs.

Initial assessment :
When admitting a patient with serious injuries, a rapid but thorough assessment is necessary. This includes securing the airway, checking the severity of injuries, detecting other associated injuries and stabilising the patient.

Airway management :
Facial burns and trauma can compromise the airway. Ensuring stable breathing, whether by intubation or emergency tracheostomy, is a priority.

Immediate wound care :
This involves cleaning, debriding if necessary, and bandaging the lesions. In the case of burns, it also includes regulating body temperature and preventing dehydration.

Reconstructive surgery :
Serious injuries may require multiple surgical interventions to repair and reconstruct facial structures. This may include skin grafts, fixation of fractures or complete reconstruction of parts of the face.

Nutritional support :
Severely burned or traumatised patients have high nutritional requirements to support healing. Appropriate nutrition, often enteral, is crucial.

Pain management :
  Burns and major trauma are extremely painful. Appropriate pain management, using a combination of drugs and other interventions, is essential for patient comfort and rehabilitation.
Physical rehabilitation and therapy :
  Beyond initial recovery, patients may require physiotherapy to regain function, as well as occupational therapy to regain daily skills.
Psychological support :
  Serious trauma can leave psychological scars just as deep as the physical ones. Psychological support, through individual or group therapy, is vital to help the patient cope with their new reality.
Social reintegration :
  Once stabilised and on the road to recovery, the patient will need help to reintegrate into society, whether by finding a job, adapting to new physical abilities, or simply returning to a normal life.
Education and prevention :
Informing patients and their families about ongoing care, potential risks and preventive measures can help prevent future incidents.

Treating extreme cases in maxillofacial surgery is a colossal task that requires a dedicated medical team and an integrative approach. Every stage, from the initial operation through to rehabilitation, is crucial to ensuring the best possible chances of recovery and quality of life for the patient.

Psychological support for the team in these intense situations

In the intense and often stressful environment of maxillofacial surgery, psychological support for the medical team is just as vital as the treatment of patients. Nurses, surgeons, anaesthetists, technicians and other healthcare professionals are faced with emotionally charged situations, complex cases and sometimes tragic outcomes. The well-being of this team is essential to ensuring quality patient care.

Recognising the signs of stress and burnout :
It is important to train team members to recognise the signs of stress, anxiety and burnout in themselves and their colleagues. These include irritability, insomnia, social withdrawal and reduced performance at work.

Post-intervention debriefing :
After particularly difficult interventions, it is beneficial to hold debriefing sessions. These meetings allow the team to express their emotions, to discuss what went well and what could have been improved.

Provision of mental health professionals :
Having a psychologist or counsellor on site or on an outpatient basis can provide a space for team members to talk about their experiences, manage their emotions and develop coping strategies.

Resilience training :
Offering workshops or training on resilience can help healthcare professionals develop techniques for coping with stress, exhaustion and possible compassion fatigue.

Encouraging physical well-being :

Physical health is closely linked to mental health. Encouraging team members to take regular breaks, eat healthily, exercise and get enough sleep can improve their ability to manage stress.

Adapted rest areas :

Provide comfortable rest areas where the team can relax, recharge their batteries and even take a nap if necessary.

Creating a culture of support :

Management and senior executives must recognise the importance of psychological support and promote a culture where seeking help is encouraged and not stigmatised.

Team building activities :

Organising regular team-building activities can help to strengthen group cohesion, improve communication and reduce stress.

Regular feedback:

Offering and soliciting regular feedback allows you to celebrate successes, recognise efforts and proactively address areas for improvement.

Taking regular leave :

Encourage the team to take time off and disconnect completely from work when they do. Regular breaks can prevent burnout.

Faced with the challenges of maxillo-facial surgery, the well-being of the team is fundamental. A team that is supported, recognised and emotionally well managed is better equipped to provide exceptional care to its patients.

Chapter 20:
THE NUANCES OF RECONSTRUCTIVE SURGERY

The main types of reconstruction

Maxillofacial surgery encompasses a diverse spectrum of procedures aimed at restoring form and function to the face and jaw. Whether following trauma, disease, tumour or congenital malformation, maxillofacial reconstruction aims to improve not only the patient's appearance, but also their quality of life by ensuring vital functions such as chewing, swallowing and phonation.

Bone reconstruction :

Bone grafting: This technique uses either the patient's own bone taken from another part of the body, donor bone or synthetic bone substitutes to reconstruct the jaw or other parts of the face.

Osteogenic distractors: Used mainly for malformations, they allow gradual extension of the bone by using the bone's natural ability to regenerate.

Soft tissue reconstruction :

Local or regional flaps: These use the tissue adjacent to the area to be reconstructed to cover a wound or an operated area.

Free flaps: This involves taking tissue from another area of the body (with its blood supply) and transplanting it into the facial area.

Temporomandibular joint (TMJ) reconstruction :

This may require implants or grafts to restore normal joint movement and eliminate pain.

- Dental and arch reconstruction :
  - Dental prostheses, dental implants and bone grafts can be used to restore functional and aesthetic teeth.
- Orthognathic surgery :
  - It aims to correct abnormalities in jaw alignment and may involve surgical repositioning of the jawbones.
- Reconstruction of the lip and palate :
  - Essential for patients with cleft lip and palate, this surgery aims to restore normal speech and swallowing function, as well as an aesthetic appearance.
- Reconstruction after tumour removal :
  - Tumours of the face and jaw may require significant removal of tissue. Reconstruction aims to restore form and function, often using a combination of techniques.
- Reconstruction of the upper aerodigestive tract :
  - After certain surgeries for tumours of the mouth, throat or larynx, reconstruction may be necessary to restore the ability to speak and swallow.
- Reconstructive rhinoplasty :
  - Used to repair or reconstruct the nose after trauma, surgery or illness.

- Auricular reconstruction :
  - This surgery can use cartilage taken from the patient to reconstruct an ear after a trauma, tumour or congenital malformation.

Reconstruction in maxillofacial surgery, although demanding, can transform patients' lives. It combines art and science, requiring the surgeon to have an in-depth understanding of anatomy, fine technical skills and aesthetic sensitivity to achieve the best results for the patient.

Managing patient expectations and families

In the world of medicine, and particularly in maxillofacial surgery, managing the expectations of patients and their families is essential. With the maxillofacial region linked to both physical appearance and essential functions such as speech, chewing and breathing, procedures can have a profound impact on patients' quality of life. Here is an in-depth exploration of how healthcare professionals can address and manage these expectations:

Preoperative education and information :
A clear understanding of the procedure, its benefits, risks and expected outcomes is essential. Providing brochures, videos or simulations can help patients visualise and understand the procedure.

Honest and open   dialogue:
It is crucial to create a space where the patient and family can express their concerns, ask questions and receive honest and clear answers.
Managing aesthetic expectations :
Maxillofacial surgery, particularly when it is aesthetic or reconstructive, requires clarification of what is aesthetically achievable, taking into account the patient's unique anatomy.
Discussion on recovery time:
Inform patients and families of the time it will take to fully recover from the operation,

including periods of swelling, pain or food restriction.

Emotional preparation :

Changes in appearance, even temporary ones, can be a source of emotional distress. Discussion and preparation for this eventuality are therefore essential.

Involvement of therapists and advisers :

In some cases, involving professionals such as psychologists or counsellors can be beneficial to help manage the emotional impact of interventions.

Regular post-operative reviews:

These appointments are used to assess progress, adjust expectations along the way and ensure that the patient and their family are supported throughout the process.

Support for families :

Relatives play a crucial role in recovery. Educating them about how they can help, what to expect, and the resources available can be just as important as supporting the patient themselves.

Support groups and testimonials :

Sometimes talking to someone who has had a similar experience can be invaluable. Support groups or patient testimonials can help put things into perspective.

Cost transparency :

A transparent discussion of costs, insurance cover and potential payment plans can reduce anxiety about the financial aspects of the operation.

The key to managing expectations lies in communication, education and ongoing support. Each patient is unique, and as such deserves a personalised approach to ensure that their expectations, and those of their loved ones, are aligned with the reality of the procedure and recovery.

Pre-operative preparation and post-operative for major operations

Maxillofacial surgery, involving vital structures of the face and head, requires meticulous preparation before and after the operation. These preparations are crucial to guarantee patient safety, minimise potential complications and ensure optimal recovery.

Pre-operative preparation :
   Full medical assessment :
         This includes blood tests, cardiac examinations and other specific assessments based on the patient's medical history.
   Specialist   consultations :
         Depending on the procedure, consultations with other specialists such as anaesthetists, orthodontists or ENT specialists may be necessary.
   Patient education :
         Inform the patient in detail about the procedure, the associated risks and post-operative expectations.
   Fasting :
         In general, patients must fast for a set period before surgery to prevent complications during anaesthesia.
   Medicines and allergies :
         Review any medication the patient is taking and adjust if necessary. It is essential to be aware of any allergies, particularly to medicines.

Cleaning the mouth :
>To minimise the risk of infection, professional dental cleaning may be recommended before certain procedures.

Post-operative planning :
>Make sure that the patient has organised transport after the operation and that he or she has planned a rest period.

Post-operative preparation :

Medical surveillance :
>Following major surgery, a period of monitoring in a post-anaesthetic unit or even an intensive care unit may be required.

Pain management :
>Prescribe and administer appropriate analgesics to control post-operative pain.

Wound care :
>Provide clear instructions on cleaning the wound, managing drains and recognising signs of infection.

Food monitoring :
>After certain operations, a liquid or soft diet may be necessary for some time.

Medicines :
>Antibiotics to prevent infection, as well as other specific drugs, may be prescribed.

Tips for reducing oedema and bruising:
>This may include elevating the head, applying ice and other methods.

Exercise and physiotherapy :
>Some patients may benefit from gentle exercise or physiotherapy to aid recovery and restore function.

Regular monitoring :
>Schedule post-operative appointments to assess recovery, discuss concerns and adjust care if necessary.

By incorporating these essential elements of pre-operative and post-operative preparation, healthcare professionals can work closely with patients to ensure a successful operation and full recovery.

Chapter 21:
THE PSYCHOLOGICAL DIMENSION
OF THE PATIENT

Maxillofacial surgery, which focuses on the face and associated structures, is not limited to simple physical reconstruction or the correction of defects. It has a profound effect on the patient's psyche, as the face is often seen as a reflection of identity and personality. Consequently, the psychological implications are at the heart of this speciality.

1. Self-perception and self-esteem :
The face is a central part of our identity. Any alteration, whether due to trauma, deformity or surgery, can change the way a patient sees and perceives themselves. Some patients may struggle with feelings of inferiority or shame about their appearance, especially in a society that places so much value on beauty and 'normality'.

2. Emotional impact of trauma :
Patients who undergo maxillofacial surgery following a trauma, whether a road accident, an assault or another cause, may also suffer from post-traumatic stress. They may relive the event, have nightmares or develop severe anxiety.

3. Fear and anxiety before surgery :
The prospect of undergoing surgery, especially on an area as visible and essential as the face, can be a source of great anxiety. Patients may fear the results, complications or pain.

4. Expectation management :
It is crucial that patients have realistic expectations of the results. Disproportionate expectations can lead to disappointment, even if the surgery is medically successful.

5. Social support and isolation :
The reactions of friends, family and strangers can greatly influence a patient's psychological well-being. Some may receive support and empathy, while others may feel isolated or misunderstood.

6. Rehabilitation and acceptance :
After surgery, the process of adapting to one's new appearance and function can be long and difficult. Some may grieve for their "old" face or struggle to accept the changes.

7. Psychological support :
Working with psychologists or therapists is often beneficial. They can offer strategies for managing anxiety, boosting self-esteem and helping with acceptance.

It is essential to recognise the depth of the psychological implications associated with maxillofacial surgery. Each patient is unique, and a holistic approach, taking into account the whole individual, is essential to ensure a complete recovery, both physically and mentally.

Understanding the psychological impact deformities and trauma

When we talk about maxillofacial surgery, we often talk about the physical aspects of the operation: reconstruction, repair and rehabilitation. However, the psychological aspect is just as crucial. Congenital malformations and accidental or intentional trauma are not only anatomical and physiological challenges, they also have profound repercussions on patients' identity, self-esteem and social integration.

1. Congenital malformations :
From an early age, a facial deformity can subject an individual to a variety of looks, comments and attitudes from those around them and from society in general. This can hinder the development of a positive body image and influence self-esteem. Children may be teased or bullied, while adults may feel judged or rejected.

2. Trauma :
Unlike malformations, trauma causes a sudden and often violent change in appearance and function. There is the physical pain, but also the emotional shock, the memory of the traumatic event and the mourning of what it was like 'before' the trauma. Survivors of accidents or assaults may experience symptoms of post-traumatic stress, such as flashbacks, insomnia or anxiety.

3. Body image :
The face is central to our non-verbal communication, our expressiveness and our identity. Any change in this area can affect the way a person perceives themselves and interacts with the world. Deformities or scars can be seen as 'marks' that attract attention, often unwanted.

4. Social repercussions :
Social interactions can be influenced by facial appearance. Some people may avoid eye contact, while others may ask intrusive questions or make inappropriate remarks. This can lead to feelings of isolation or social withdrawal.

5. Resilience and healing :
Each individual is unique in their ability to cope with and overcome the psychological challenges associated with malformations and trauma. Some find strength in their

experience, turning it into motivation to help others or raise public awareness. Others may require more intensive psychological support to get them through.

Although maxillofacial surgery procedures can greatly improve appearance and function, it is imperative to understand and address the profound psychological implications. Comprehensive and holistic care, encompassing both physical and emotional needs, will ensure the best results and true healing for the patient.

Patient support and counselling

Maxillofacial surgery, although essentially medical and surgical in nature, has a profoundly emotional and psychological impact on patients. The face is our calling card, the primary image we project to the world. Any operation or change in this area can therefore upset our self-perception, our self-esteem and the way others perceive us. Support and counselling are therefore crucial in helping patients through this ordeal, whether they are undergoing reconstructive surgery after a trauma or an elective procedure for aesthetic or functional reasons.

1. Preparing for the operation :
Before the operation, patients often have concerns, hopes and expectations. Psychological support allows these concerns to be addressed, realistic expectations to be set and helps the patient to consider the various possible outcomes.

2. Managing post-operative emotions :
After surgery, it is common to experience a range of emotions, from euphoria to depression and uncertainty. Counselling can help the patient navigate through this

emotional turmoil, managing post-operative pain, changes in appearance and possible complications.

3. Social rehabilitation :
Returning to everyday life with a face that has been altered, even slightly, can be unsettling. Patients may fear judgement, stigmatisation or intrusive questions. Therapists can provide tools and strategies for coping with these social interactions.

4. Support for the family :
The patient's loved ones play an essential role in the healing process. They can also benefit from information and counselling sessions to help them understand the surgical process, post-operative expectations and how best to support their loved one.

5. Support groups :
Sharing your experience with others who have been through similar circumstances can be liberating. Support groups offer a safe space to share, listen and learn from each other.

6. Long-term support :
Even after physical healing, emotional scars can persist. Long-term counselling sessions can help address these underlying issues, giving patients a space to talk about their concerns and find solutions.

7. Resources and references :
Healthcare professionals must have a list of resources, ranging from specialist clinical psychologists to support groups, to meet patients' specific needs.

Support and counselling for maxillofacial surgery patients are essential aspects of the care process. Recognising and responding to patients' emotional and psychological needs can greatly enhance their satisfaction, recovery and overall quality of life.

Managing dysmorphophobia

Dysmorphophobia, also known as body dysmorphic disorder (BDD), is an obsessive preoccupation with a perceived defect in physical appearance, often imaginary or minimal. In the field of maxillofacial surgery, these patients may seek multiple surgical interventions to correct these 'defects', without ever being satisfied with the results. Managing these patients is a particular challenge that requires a multidisciplinary approach.

1. Early identification :
The first steps in helping patients with CDT are to identify their concerns and understand their perceptions. A patient may be fixated on a minor detail, have unrealistic expectations or express persistent dissatisfaction with previous surgeries.

2. Psychological assessment :
Before considering any surgical intervention, it is essential to carry out a thorough psychological assessment. This will determine whether the patient is suffering from dysmorphophobia or another underlying disorder.

3. Education and advice :
It is crucial to educate patients about the nature of their disorder. They need to understand that surgery is not a solution and may even exacerbate their concerns.

4. Refusal of surgery :
In many cases, the best approach is to refuse to perform cosmetic surgery on a patient with DCT. Although this may seem counter-intuitive, it is in the patient's best interest, as further surgery can worsen the condition.

5. Therapeutic approach :
Cognitive-behavioural therapies have been shown to be effective in treating CDD. They help patients to recognise and change their negative thought patterns and self-destructive behaviours.

6. Medication :
Some antidepressants, particularly selective serotonin reuptake inhibitors (SSRIs), may be beneficial for patients with CDD.
7. Regular monitoring :
It is important to ensure regular follow-up with patients to monitor their psychological state, even if they have chosen not to undergo surgery.

8. Multidisciplinary collaboration :
Working closely with psychologists, psychiatrists and other mental health professionals is essential to providing comprehensive care.

9. Support and therapy groups :
Encouraging patients to join support groups or group therapy sessions can help them feel less isolated and learn from the experiences of others.

10. Educating professionals :
Training maxillo-facial surgeons and other medical professionals to recognise the signs of CDT can help ensure patients are managed appropriately.

Although maxillofacial surgery can offer excellent aesthetic and functional results, it is not always the appropriate response for patients with dysmorphophobia. An empathetic, informed and multidisciplinary approach is essential to ensure the well-being of these patients.

Chapter 22:
MAXILLO-FACIAL SURGERY AND ONCOLOGY

Patient care with cancer

The management of cancer patients in maxillofacial surgery is a multifaceted challenge that requires not only technical expertise but also a holistic, patient-centred approach. Cancer of the maxillofacial region, which encompasses various tumours of the mouth, throat, nose, sinuses and other adjacent areas, requires careful planning and interdisciplinary collaboration.

1. Diagnosis and assessment :
It all starts with a thorough clinical assessment. Imaging techniques, such as X-rays, CT scans and MRIs, play a crucial role in determining the extent of the tumour. Biopsy confirms the diagnosis.

2. Staging :
It is essential to determine the stage of the cancer, as this will guide treatment decisions. Staging takes into account the size of the tumour, its spread to neighbouring structures and the possible presence of metastases.

3. Treatment planning :
Once a diagnosis has been made, a multidisciplinary team meets to draw up a treatment plan. This team may include maxillofacial surgeons, oncologists, radiologists, pathologists, nutritionists, speech therapists and other specialists.

4. Surgery :
Depending on the type, location and stage of the cancer, surgery may be recommended to remove the tumour. In

some cases, reconstruction may be necessary, using grafts or flaps of tissue from other parts of the body.

5. Radiotherapy and chemotherapy :
These treatments may be offered before or after surgery, or even in the absence of surgery, depending on the type and stage of the cancer.

6. Rehabilitation :
Rehabilitation is often a crucial aspect following treatment for maxillofacial cancer. This can include physiotherapy to restore mobility, speech therapy for speech and swallowing, and dental or facial prostheses if necessary.

7. Long-term follow-up :
Regular monitoring is crucial for the early detection of any recurrence or complication. This involves regular clinical examinations and imaging.

8. Psychosocial support :
The diagnosis of cancer and its treatment can have a significant emotional impact. Psychological support, whether through individual counselling or support groups, is vital.

9. Education and prevention :
It is essential to educate patients about the signs of recurrence and modifiable risk factors, such as smoking or alcohol consumption.

10. Search and advanced :
The treatment of maxillofacial cancers is constantly evolving thanks to research. Patients need to be kept informed of the latest advances and, in some cases, can benefit from clinical trials.

The management of cancer patients in maxillofacial surgery is a multidimensional journey that goes far beyond the simple excision of a tumour. It requires a comprehensive and well-coordinated approach to ensure not only survival, but also the patient's quality of life.

Palliative care management in maxillo-facial surgery

Palliative care is an approach that aims to improve the quality of life of patients and their families faced with problems associated with a life-threatening illness. In maxillofacial surgery, this approach is essential for patients with advanced tumours or for those who are not candidates for curative treatment. This care focuses on the prevention and relief of suffering, whether physical, psychological, social or spiritual.

1. Overall assessment :
First and foremost, a full assessment of the patient is required. This covers not only the medical aspect, but also the patient's psychological, social and spiritual needs.

2. Pain management :
Pain is a frequent symptom and can be particularly excruciating in maxillofacial conditions. It may arise from the tumour itself or from surgical procedures. A combination of analgesics, including opioids, may be required.

3. Wound care :
Tumour wounds or post-surgical wounds may require specialised care, particularly to control infection, remove debris and promote healing.

4. Nutrition :
Problems with chewing, swallowing or excessive saliva secretion can impair a patient's ability to eat. Nutritional

strategies, including the placement of a feeding tube, may be necessary.

5. Communication :
Tumours or surgery can affect a patient's ability to speak. Speech and language therapists and other specialists can help to improve speech.
communication.

6. Psychological support :
The diagnosis and progression of the disease can have a considerable emotional impact. Psychotherapists, counsellors and support groups can help.

7. Spiritual aspects :
For many patients, illness raises questions of meaning, value and spirituality. Chaplains or other spiritual advisers can offer invaluable support.

8. Advance planning :
It is crucial to discuss the patient's wishes regarding future care, including advance directives and power of attorney for healthcare.

9. End of life :
When the end of life approaches, particular attention must be paid to the patient's comfort. This may mean reducing or modifying treatment, administering medication to relieve discomfort and providing emotional support for the patient and their family.

10. Family support :
The family plays a crucial role in palliative care. They need support to understand the illness, manage stress and bereavement, and make informed decisions.

Palliative care in maxillofacial surgery focuses on the patient's overall well-being, going beyond simple symptom management. It requires a holistic and interdisciplinary approach to ensure the patient's comfort and dignity at every stage of their illness.

Working with the oncology team

In the world of medicine, where specialisation has become the norm, interdisciplinary collaboration is more essential than ever. At the heart of this dynamic is the interaction between the maxillofacial surgery nurse and the oncology team. This alliance is of crucial importance when it comes to treating malignant diseases of the maxillofacial region, where the stakes are often twofold: eradicating the cancer while preserving function and aesthetics as far as possible.

When a patient is diagnosed with maxillofacial cancer, the nurse is often the first healthcare professional they turn to. In addition to primary care, the nurse plays a central role in coordinating the various specialists who will be involved throughout the patient's course of treatment. Chemotherapy, radiotherapy or surgery, sometimes combined, are common treatment modalities, with each stage requiring separate preparation and follow-up.

The role of the nurse goes well beyond the clinical setting. It is the nurse who often helps the patient to understand the complexity of the treatments proposed by the oncologist, radiologist or maxillo-facial surgeon. What's more, as the bridge between the patient and the medical team, the nurse translates the patient's concerns and needs to the team, ensuring that every decision taken is truly patient-centred.

But this collaboration with the oncology team does not stop at the end of treatment. Post-treatment monitoring is essential to detect any recurrence or late complications.

Here again, the nurse is on the front line, regularly monitoring the patient, assessing the quality of his or her recovery, and reporting any worrying signs to the oncology team.

In the often tumultuous journey of the maxillofacial cancer patient, the nurse is much more than just a care provider. He or she is the guardian of continuity of care, an invaluable intermediary between the patient and the oncology team, and a pillar on which the patient can rely at every stage of his or her recovery.

Chapter 23:
IMPLANTOLOGY AND PROSTHODONTICS

Basic principles of implantology

Implantology is a speciality of dental surgery that focuses on placing implants in the jaw to replace one or more missing teeth. Much more than just a cosmetic solution, dental implants help restore chewing function and prevent many of the complications associated with tooth loss. Let's delve into the fundamentals of this fascinating discipline.

1. Understanding Dental Implants
A dental implant is essentially a titanium screw inserted into the jawbone, serving as an artificial root to which a crown, bridge or prosthesis can be attached. Titanium is chosen for its biocompatibility, allowing perfect osseointegration with the surrounding bone tissue.

2. Osseointegration: an intimate union
The success of an implant lies in its ability to fuse with the jawbone, a process known as osseointegration. This solid fusion is essential to ensure the implant's stability and enable it to withstand the forces exerted during chewing.

3. Pre-implant assessment
Before an implant is placed, a thorough assessment is required. This includes radiographic examinations to assess the quantity and quality of the bone, determine the optimal location for the implant and identify any contraindications.

4. Surgical techniques
The implant procedure varies according to the patient's needs. It can be immediate, where the implant is placed

immediately after a tooth extraction, or delayed, allowing the extraction area to heal before the implant is placed.

5. Implant-supported prostheses
Once osseointegration has taken place, a prosthesis is attached to the implant. This may be a crown for a single tooth, a bridge for several teeth or a complete prosthesis to replace all the teeth.

6. Care of Implants
Although implants are resistant to decay, the surrounding tissue is susceptible to infection if proper oral hygiene is not maintained. It is therefore crucial to adopt a rigorous cleaning routine and to consult a dental health professional regularly.

7. Developments and innovations
As technology advances, implantology is undergoing constant innovation. These include less invasive techniques, improved materials, and even the possibility of using 3D imaging for precise surgical planning.

Implantology has transformed the way we approach tooth loss, offering a durable and functional solution for many patients. Beyond technique, implant success is based on a thorough understanding of anatomy, careful planning and a commitment to clinical excellence.

Post-operative management of patients with implants

The period following implant surgery is crucial to the success of the operation. Appropriate post-operative management is essential to guarantee optimal healing, avoid complications and ensure the longevity of the implant. Here's a detailed look at this essential phase.

1. First 48 hours: Reduction of Inflammation and Pain
After surgery, it is common to experience swelling, bruising or tenderness around the surgical area. Taking anti-inflammatories and analgesics, as prescribed by the surgeon, will help to control these symptoms. Applying cold compresses can also help reduce inflammation.

2. Oral hygiene: Gentle and precise
It is essential to keep your mouth clean to avoid infections. However, in the days following the operation, brushing directly on the surgical site should be avoided so as not to disturb the healing area. The use of an antiseptic mouthwash may be recommended.

3. Diet: Gentle and nutritious
In the week following surgery, it is advisable to adopt a soft diet to avoid any pressure or trauma on the implant. Soups, purées, yoghurts and compotes are good choices. It is also best to avoid extremely hot drinks.

4. Post-operative follow-up: guaranteeing a smooth recovery
Post-operative appointments are generally scheduled to check on the state of healing, ensure that there is no infection and assess the osseointegration of the implant. These appointments are essential to anticipate and manage any possible complications.

5. Implant integration : Patience and precision
Depending on the type and location of the implant, as well as the patient's general health, the osseointegration period may vary. It is essential to follow the surgeon's recommendations during this waiting phase to ensure solid fusion between the implant and the bone.

6. Prosthesis: the final touch
Once the implant is securely anchored, a dental prosthesis (crown, bridge or other) is fixed to it. The care and hygiene

of this prosthesis are just as essential to guarantee the durability of the whole.

7. Long-term life with implants
With the right care, an implant can last a lifetime. This requires rigorous oral hygiene, regular check-ups with the dentist and attention to any changes or discomfort experienced.

The post-operative management of patients with implants is a shared responsibility between the healthcare professional and the patient. Together, they can ensure that the healing process runs smoothly and that the implant performs its function optimally.

Working with prosthodontists and dental technicians

Maxillofacial surgery, while a distinct and complex speciality in its own right, often works in close collaboration with other dental specialities, particularly prosthodontics. The symbiosis between the maxillo-facial surgeon, the prosthodontist and the dental technician is essential to ensure the best results for the patient.

1. The role of each: complementarity and specialisation
The maxillo-facial surgeon focuses on surgical procedures relating to the bone structure of the face and jaw, while the prosthodontist specialises in the design and fitting of dental prostheses. The dental technician designs and manufactures these prosthetic devices in the laboratory to the prosthodontist's specifications.

2. Joint planning : The key to success
The success of any treatment, whether a full restoration or an implant, often depends on careful planning. Before any

operation, the surgeon, prosthodontist and dental technician meet to draw up a plan based on the patient's anatomy and functional and aesthetic needs.

3. Regular Communication: Ensuring Monitoring and Optimisation
Constant updates between these professionals ensure that each stage is carried out with precision. The dental technician may need clarification on the dimensions or materials of a prosthesis, while the prosthodontist and surgeon can discuss the best surgical options for the planned prosthesis.

4. Continuing education: Evolving together
Dental care technology and techniques are evolving rapidly. As a result, all three players need to undergo regular training to stay up to date and offer the best possible care. Joint workshops and seminars can strengthen mutual understanding and refine collaborative techniques.

5. The Patient at the Centre: A Holistic Approach
The collaboration between the surgeon, prosthodontist and dental technician enables a patient-centred approach. Together, they can address the whole situation, from surgery to rehabilitation, ensuring that the patient is well informed and comfortable at every stage.

Close collaboration between the maxillo-facial surgeon, the prosthodontist and the dental technician is fundamental to quality dental care. Each brings their unique expertise to the table, and together they work in synergy to deliver optimal results for the patient. This collaborative dynamic is at the heart of modern medicine, where multidisciplinarity is more than ever a guarantee of quality and excellence.

Chapter 24:
ADVANCED TECHNIQUES
AND EMERGING TECHNOLOGIES

Computer-assisted surgery

The integration of computer technology into the medical world has created a silent but profound revolution. Maxillofacial surgery, in particular, has benefited from the precision, efficiency and visualisation advantages offered by computer-assisted surgery (CAD).

1. The Emergence of CAD : From Timid Beginnings to Technological Revolution
The first forays into computer-aided surgery were marked by the use of basic software to facilitate the visualisation of anatomical structures. Now, with advanced programmes and interactive interfaces, surgeons can simulate, plan and perform operations with unrivalled precision.

2. Benefits of Precision: Reducing Risk and Optimising Outcomes
One of CAD's greatest assets is its ability to provide three-dimensional visualisation of anatomical structures, enabling surgeons to anticipate potential challenges and adjust their approach. This often results in shorter operations, fewer complications and a faster recovery for the patient.

3. Pre-operative planning: a glimpse before the incision
Simulation tools allow surgeons to visualise expected outcomes and discuss options with patients. By superimposing X-ray images and three-dimensional scans, CAD creates a detailed map of the surgical area, providing an unprecedented overview of the procedure.

4. Surgical Navigation in Real Time: A Compass for the Surgeon
During surgery, computer-assisted surgery acts as a navigation system, guiding the surgeon through the procedure. This can be particularly useful during complex operations or in anatomical areas that are difficult to access.

5. Merging with Other Technologies: Robotics and Advanced Imaging
CAD is not an isolated technology. It integrates perfectly with other advances, such as robot-assisted surgery and innovative imaging techniques. This synergy multiplies the benefits for both patient and practitioner.

6. The Future of Computer-Aided Surgery: Towards New Horizons
As technology continues to evolve, CAD is becoming increasingly sophisticated. The incorporation of augmented reality, artificial intelligence and tactile interfaces is paving the way for ever more precise and individualised interventions.

Computer-assisted surgery is a powerful tool that, in the hands of a skilled surgeon, can transform and enhance the landscape of maxillofacial surgery. It symbolises the fusion of the medical art with technological advances, offering optimal patient care while pushing the boundaries of what is surgically possible.

Grafting techniques and transplantation

When it comes to maxillofacial surgery, grafting and transplantation techniques play an essential role in the restoration and reconstruction of tissue defects or loss. They are often necessary to restore form, function and sometimes aesthetics to patients affected by trauma, malformations, tumours or other conditions.

1. *The need for grafts and transplants:*
Whether following tumour resection, traumatic injury or to correct a malformation, grafts are used to make up for a lack of tissue, while transplants aim to replace a diseased organ or tissue with a healthy equivalent.

2. Types of Graft in Maxillofacial Surgery:
- **Bone graft:** Used to fill bone defects, it can come from the patient himself (autograft), from a donor (allograft), or be synthetic. Common donor sites include the skull, hip or tibia.
- **Skin grafting:** For skin defects, sections of skin can be removed and transplanted. Depending on the thickness of the skin removed, these are referred to as total or partial grafts.
- **Soft tissue graft:** This involves muscle, cartilage or other soft tissue.

3. *Advanced transplants:*
Developments in medical techniques have enabled partial or complete facial transplants, making it possible for severely affected patients to recover facial function and appearance.

4. *Anastomosis techniques:*
A crucial aspect of grafts and transplants is the need to reconnect blood vessels and sometimes nerves to ensure the viability of the grafted tissue. Surgeons use microsurgery for these delicate anastomoses, ensuring good blood flow and functionality.

5. *Rejection and immunosuppression:*
One of the major concerns after transplantation, particularly with allografts, is rejection. To reduce this risk,

patients often require immunosuppressive treatment, which has its own challenges and side effects.

6. Future and potential:
With advances in tissue bioengineering and the advent of biological 3D printing, future grafts could be 'grown' in the laboratory from the patient's own cells, eliminating the risk of rejection.

Grafting and transplantation techniques in maxillofacial surgery are constantly evolving, offering hope and solutions to patients facing complex medical challenges. Through a combination of surgical skill, advanced technology and tailored post-operative care, the lives of many patients are transformed, enabling them to regain not only their physical fitness, but also their self-confidence.

The promise of robotic surgery

At the intersection of technology and medicine, robotic surgery is emerging as a genuine revolution, promising to push back the limits of what traditional surgery can achieve, particularly in areas as delicate as maxillofacial surgery.

1. Greater precision:
One of the major advantages of robotic surgery is its unrivalled precision. Robots are equipped with articulated arms that can perform very precise movements, eliminating the natural tremors of the human hand. This is particularly beneficial for operations requiring millimetre-level accuracy.

2. Access to difficult areas:
The slim, articulated design of the robotic arms allows access to areas that are difficult to reach with the human

hand, minimising incisions and therefore post-operative scarring.

3. Reduced surgeon fatigue:
Performing surgery, especially of long duration, can be exhausting for the surgeon. Robots, once correctly positioned, can maintain their position without weakening, allowing the surgeon to concentrate on the precise aspect of the operation.

4. Improved vision:
With the use of high-definition cameras and magnification systems, surgeons have a clear, enlarged view of the surgical field, which is essential for complex anatomical areas of the face.

5. Reduced recovery time:
Thanks to smaller, more precise incisions, patients often benefit from faster healing, less post-operative pain and a shorter hospital stay.

6. Training and telesurgery:
Robotic surgery paves the way for telesurgery, where an expert can operate remotely, and improved training for future surgeons through virtual reality simulations.

7. Potential for innovation:
The fusion of robotic surgery with other technologies, such as real-time imaging, artificial intelligence, or 3D printing, could further expand the field of possibilities in maxillofacial surgery.

However, despite its promise, robotic surgery is not without its challenges. Its high cost, the need for specialist training, and the ethical debates surrounding the use of robots in medicine are all obstacles to be overcome.

Robotic surgery represents an exciting step in the evolution of maxillofacial surgery. As techniques are perfected and technology becomes more accessible, it could well transform the way surgery is performed, offering better outcomes for patients and more advanced tools for surgeons.

Chapter 25:
MANAGEMENT
RARE COMPLICATIONS

Neurological complications

When it comes to maxillofacial surgery, it is essential to understand the anatomical complexity of this region. Not only is the face the site of our visual identity, it is also a region rich in nerve structures. Neurological complications can arise during surgery, affecting not only function but also the patient's quality of life.

1. Nature of complications :
Neurological complications in maxillofacial surgery may be temporary or permanent and may result from trauma, surgical incisions, compression or infection.

2. Sensory nerves :
One of the most common complications involves the inferior alveolar nerve, which gives sensation to the lower lip and chin. Damage to this nerve can lead to paresthesia, a sensation of tingling or numbness. Similarly, the lingual nerve, which is responsible for tongue sensation, can be affected during certain operations.

3. Motor nerves :
The facial nerve is the main motor nerve of the face. Its damage can lead to facial paralysis, affecting facial expression, eyelid closure and speech. Although such complications are rare, they can have devastating consequences for the patient.

4. Post-operative complications :
Haematomas or oedema may compress the nerves, causing temporary deficits. Infections can also lead to

neurological complications if they spread to nerve structures.

5. Management of complications :
Treatment of neurological complications depends on the cause and severity. Some nerve deficits may resolve over time, while others require intervention to decompress a nerve or treat an infection. Rehabilitation, such as facial physiotherapy, can be useful for patients with motor deficits.

6. Prevention :
The best way to manage neurological complications is to prevent them. This involves careful surgical planning, a good knowledge of anatomy, the use of advanced imaging tools and precise surgical technique.

7. Importance of communication :
It is crucial to inform patients of the potential risks associated with surgery. Open communication helps to manage expectations and ensure that the patient is well informed before giving consent.

Although maxillofacial surgery is generally safe, neurological complications can occur. A thorough understanding of anatomy, meticulous surgical technique and appropriate management of complications can help minimise these risks and ensure the best outcome for the patient.

Vascular complications and haemorrhage

Maxillofacial surgery, because of its proximity to important vascular structures, presents a risk of vascular and haemorrhagic complications. Understanding these complications and knowing how to manage them is essential to ensure patient safety.

1. The vascular tissue of the face :
The face is irrigated by a rich vascular network, mainly by the external carotid arteries and their branches. Any incision or manipulation in this region requires special care to avoid damaging these vessels.

2. Vascular complications :
These may take the form of thrombosis, embolism or aneurysm. These complications may result from vascular lesions during the operation or post-operatively.

3. Haemorrhage :
Haemorrhage is one of the most common complications in maxillofacial surgery. It can occur during or after surgery. Severe haemorrhage can lead to life-threatening haemorrhagic shock.

4. Prevention and management of bleeding :
   - **During the operation**: Good visibility of the operating field, the use of precise instruments and careful coagulation of the blood vessels all help to minimise the risk of haemorrhage.
   - **Post-operative**: Close monitoring is essential to detect signs of haemorrhage early, such as the formation of a haematoma, increasing pain or low blood pressure. Treatment may require surgery to stop the bleeding and drain the haematoma.

5. Other complications linked to haemorrhage :
   - **Haematoma**: Accumulation of blood in a surgical area. It may require surgical evacuation if it is large or if it exerts pressure on vital structures.
   - **Delayed haemorrhage**: This can occur several days after surgery, often as a result of inflammation or infection.

6. *Importance of preparation:*
Before any surgery, it is crucial to obtain a full medical history to identify patients at increased risk of bleeding, such as those on anticoagulants, or with bleeding disorders.

7. *Collaboration with other specialists:*
In complex cases, collaboration with vascular specialists or interventional radiologists may be necessary to assess, prevent and manage vascular complications.

Maxillofacial surgery, despite its challenges, remains a specialty where, with proper training and meticulous attention to detail, the risks of vascular and haemorrhagic complications can be significantly reduced. Clear communication with the patient about the risks and careful preparation are essential to ensure optimal results.

Management of atypical cases

The field of maxillofacial surgery, while extremely specialised, encompasses a wide variety of cases, some routine and others distinctly atypical. The latter often pose a challenge to the medical team in terms of diagnosis, planning and surgical intervention.

1. *Recognising atypicality :*
This is the first challenge. An atypical case may present with unusual symptoms, rare clinical presentations or complex co-morbidities that alter the traditional clinical picture. Sometimes it is a combination of factors that makes a case unique.

2. *Diagnostic approach :*
An accurate diagnosis is the cornerstone of the management of any medical case. In atypical situations,

this may require additional investigations, the use of advanced diagnostic tests or even consultation with experts in related fields.

3. Surgical planning :
An atypical case may often require an adapted or personalised surgical approach. This could include the use of non-traditional techniques or equipment, or the modification of standard procedures to suit the specific situation.

4. Managing expectations :
Patients with atypical cases may have different expectations regarding results, recovery time and possible complications. Clear communication is essential to ensure understanding and informed consent.

5. Interdisciplinary support :
Atypical cases often benefit from interdisciplinary management, where various specialists work together to provide the best possible care. For example, a patient with a complex congenital malformation might require the expertise of an orthodontist, a plastic surgeon and a maxillo-facial surgeon.

6. Post-operative review:
Atypical cases may have unpredictable post-operative courses. Close monitoring, regular check-ups and, occasionally, additional interventions may be required to ensure optimal recovery.

7. Ongoing training and knowledge sharing:
Every atypical case offers an opportunity to learn. It is essential for maxillo-facial surgeons to keep abreast of the latest research, techniques and technologies. In addition, sharing experiences with the medical community can help other professionals facing similar situations.

While atypical cases in maxillofacial surgery can present additional challenges, they also offer a unique opportunity for professional growth, innovation and improved patient care. A holistic, interdisciplinary and patient-centred approach is the key to success in managing these unique situations.

Chapter 26:
LIFE AFTER SURGERY:
LONG-TERM FOLLOW-UP

Establish regular monitoring protocols

Post-operative follow-up is a crucial element of care in maxillofacial surgery. It not only ensures correct healing, but also identifies complications early on, optimises aesthetic and functional results and strengthens the relationship of trust between the patient and the medical team. The implementation of structured and systematic follow-up protocols is therefore essential.

1. Objectives of follow-up :
The main objectives of regular follow-up are to assess recovery, detect any complications, ensure patient satisfaction and make adjustments or additional interventions if necessary.

2. First post-operative consultation :
This consultation generally takes place a few days after the operation. It provides an opportunity to assess the initial healing, to ensure that the patient is following the post-operative instructions, and to answer any questions or concerns.

3. Frequency of visits :
The frequency of visits depends on the nature of the operation. Some surgeries require weekly visits initially, then monthly, while others may only require one or two check-ups.

4. Specific assessments :
Depending on the type of operation, specific assessments

may be required, such as X-rays, scans, muscle function tests or aesthetic assessments.

5. Duration of monitoring :
The follow-up period varies depending on the procedure. Some procedures, such as dental extractions, may require a follow-up of a few weeks to a few months, while more complex operations, such as facial reconstruction, may require a follow-up of several years.

6. Communication with other health professionals :
Maxillo-facial surgeons often work in collaboration with other specialists. Regular and comprehensive communication with these professionals is essential for holistic patient care.

7. Records management :
It is essential to maintain accurate and detailed medical records for each patient, including notes of each consultation, photographs, test results and any other relevant information.

8. Ongoing patient education:
Follow-up is also an opportunity for ongoing patient education on home care, prevention of complications and general health promotion.

9. Review of protocols :
Follow-up protocols should be reviewed regularly to ensure that they reflect current best practice and meet the changing needs of patients.
Implementing regular follow-up protocols in maxillofacial surgery is crucial to optimising patient outcomes and minimising complications. A systematic, individualised and patient-focused approach will ensure quality care and satisfactory results.

Managing long-term problems
or late complications

Maxillofacial surgery, despite its complexity and precise level of intervention, is not exempt from long-term complications or late problems. Whether it's an unexpected after-effect or a side-effect of an operation, long-term follow-up is crucial to ensure the patient's well-being and the success of the procedure.

1. Nature of long-term complications :
Complications may vary depending on the nature of the initial operation. They may include deformities, joint dysfunction, chronic pain, hypertrophic scars or occlusion problems.

2. Regular follow-up :
Even after the immediate post-operative period, it is vital to have follow-up consultations to monitor the healing progress and ensure that no latent problems arise.

3. Ongoing rehabilitation :
Some patients may require long-term rehabilitation, particularly to regain normal muscle function, or to manage persistent pain. Collaboration with physiotherapists, speech therapists and other specialists may be necessary.

4. Repeat surgery :
In some cases, unfortunately, a secondary operation may be necessary to correct problems that have only manifested themselves in the long term.

5. Patient advice and education :
It is essential to inform the patient of the signs of potential complications so that they can recognise them and seek advice quickly. These may include pain, changes in sensation or mobility, or visual changes.

6. Psychological management :
The long-term effects of maxillofacial surgery are not just physical. The psychological component can be just as important. Some patients may have difficulty adapting to their new appearance or dealing with the trauma of a major operation. Psychological support can be crucial in these cases.

7. Prevention :
The best way to manage long-term complications is to prevent them. Careful surgical planning, impeccable technique and rigorous post-operative follow-up can significantly reduce the risk of late problems.

8. Research and feedback :
Finally, in order to continually improve procedures and techniques, it is essential to collect data on long-term complications. This feedback can help refine surgical techniques, improve surgeon training and guide future research in the field.
The management of long-term problems or late complications in maxillofacial surgery requires a comprehensive approach that encompasses medical follow-up, rehabilitation, psychological support and patient education. A proactive, patient-centred approach will ensure the best possible results and the long-term well-being of patients.

Psychological support and social reintegration

Maxillofacial surgery, as a discipline, is not limited to the physical and functional restoration of the face and mouth. It also has profound ramifications for the patient's psyche, as the face is a reflection of identity and self-esteem. After an operation, a patient may face a myriad of psychological and social challenges, which is why it is so important to provide comprehensive care to help them reintegrate into society.

1. The psychological impact of surgery :
A physical change, even if desired or necessary, can lead to a period of adjustment for the patient. Issues relating to identity, self-esteem and self-perception may be disrupted, leading to feelings of sadness, confusion or even grief.

2. Therapeutic support :
Therapy with a psychologist or psychiatrist may be essential to help the patient navigate this difficult period. This help can address issues such as depression, anxiety or post-traumatic stress.

3. Support groups:
Support groups provide a space where patients can share their experiences, learn from each other and support each other. These interactions can often help to normalise their feelings and reassure them that they are not alone in their struggle.

4. Preparation for social reintegration :
The reactions of others to the patient's post-operative appearance may vary. Some patients may fear judgement, stigmatisation or isolation. Information sessions, coaching or social simulation can help prepare the patient for these interactions.

5. Rehabilitation programmes :
Tailored programmes to help the patient regain vocational skills, return to work or resume their usual activities may be beneficial.

6. The patient's entourage :
It is essential to involve the patient's family and close friends in the recovery process. Supporting them and

educating them about what to expect and how to help the patient can make all the difference.

7. Acceptance and self-esteem:
It is crucial to work with the patient to help them accept and love their new appearance, recognise their intrinsic value and boost their self-confidence.

8. Long-term follow-up :
Social reintegration and psychological support do not stop once the patient leaves hospital. Regular follow-up, psychological check-ups and checkpoints can help to identify and deal with any emerging problems.
Maxillofacial surgery does not stop in the operating theatre. To ensure true healing and successful reintegration, it is essential to take into account the patient's psychological and social well-being. By adopting a holistic, patient-centred approach, healthcare professionals can truly transform the lives of those they care for.

Chapter 27:
PATIENT SAFETY
AND RISK MANAGEMENT

Security protocols
in the operating theatre

The operating theatre is the scene of complex and precise medical interventions, particularly in the field of maxillofacial surgery. In this environment, patient safety remains the paramount concern, making strict, well-defined protocols essential.

From the moment patients enter the room, every step is orchestrated to eliminate any possibility of error. The process of checking patient identities is meticulous, ensuring that the right procedure is carried out on the right patient. Once confirmed, the procedure area is prepared and disinfected with the utmost care, while ensuring patient comfort.

The equipment used is scrupulously checked. From sterilised instruments to life-support machines, each tool has its own safety protocol. The correct operation of anaesthesia machines, for example, is essential to ensure a smooth operation.
Communication is the linchpin of safety in the operating theatre. The surgical team engages in constant dialogue, sharing crucial information in real time. Even before the first incision, the surgeon confirms the procedure to be followed, ensuring that every member of the team is aligned with expectations and responsibilities.

During the operation, the patient is constantly monitored. Vital signs are continuously monitored, and any abnormality, however minor, is immediately reported and treated. This means that any unforeseen event can be anticipated and managed effectively.

The operating theatre is also a place where hygiene is paramount. Asepsis protocols are rigorously applied to avoid any contamination or infection. Team members are dressed in sterile garments and follow strict hand-washing and glove-wearing rules.

Finally, after the operation, the patient is carefully transferred to a recovery room where he or she is closely monitored, ensuring a safe recovery from anaesthesia. The surgeon then reviews the details of the procedure with the patient and their family, ensuring that everything is understood and that the post-operative care plan is clearly established.

This constant concern for safety, anchored in every stage of the operation, reflects the unfailing commitment of maxillofacial surgery to the well-being of its patients.

Incident management and adverse events

Maxillo-facial surgery, like all medical specialities, is not immune to incidents or adverse events. These situations, although rare, require proactive, methodical and transparent management to ensure patient safety and maintain public confidence in the healthcare system.
When an incident occurs, the immediate priority is to ensure the patient's stability and well-being. The medical team deploys all the resources and skills necessary to stabilise the situation, correct the anomaly and prevent any further damage.

Following the incident, an internal investigation is systematically launched to determine the causes. This approach is part of a drive to continuously improve the quality of care. The professionals involved are encouraged to share their observations and analyses without fear of reprisal, because it is by identifying errors that they can be avoided in the future.

A key element in incident management is transparent communication with patients and their families. They must be informed of the nature of the incident, the measures taken to remedy it and the possible consequences for their health. This honest and open approach strengthens the relationship of trust between the patient and the healthcare team.

At the same time, reporting protocols are in place to alert the relevant regulatory and professional bodies. These reports are essential for monitoring trends, identifying recurring risks and developing prevention strategies on a national scale.

Once the analysis is complete, the lessons learned from the incident are incorporated into the ongoing training of our teams. Workshops, simulations and training courses are organised to ensure that each professional is well equipped to anticipate and manage this type of situation.

Finally, the implementation of corrective measures is often based on a multidisciplinary approach. Whether it's adjusting protocols, updating equipment or reviewing work methods, every change is designed to improve the safety and quality of interventions.

Incident management in maxillo-facial surgery is therefore a structured, patient-centred and forward-looking process. It reflects the specialty's commitment to providing the highest quality care, even in the most unforeseen circumstances.

Promoting a culture of safety within the team

In the dynamic and often unpredictable world of maxillofacial surgery, patient safety is paramount. More than just a series of protocols and guidelines, safety is a state of mind, a culture. Promoting this culture within a medical team requires a multifactorial approach, centred on collaboration, training and empowerment.

Firstly, it is essential to recognise that each member of the team, whether surgeon, nurse, anaesthetist or technician, brings a unique expertise and perspective. Fostering an environment where every voice is heard and valued encourages feedback, particularly on any concerns or anomalies. The aim is to create a climate of trust where the fear of reprisals or judgement does not hinder communication.

Ongoing training is also a pillar of this culture. Medical advances, new technologies and feedback from previous incidents must be regularly incorporated into training programmes. Simulations, practical workshops and real-life case reviews help to prepare the team for day-to-day challenges, while reinforcing safety reflexes.

Accountability is another key element. Each member of the team must understand their role in the safety chain and be aware of the impact of their actions on the patient and their colleagues. Evaluation and feedback systems, whether formal or informal, can help to reinforce this individual and collective responsibility.

In addition, the introduction of checklists, largely inspired by aviation, has proved effective in ensuring that all the critical stages of a procedure are followed. As well as being practical tools, these checklists are also constant reminders of the importance of rigour and systematisation when it comes to safety.

It is also essential to celebrate successes and improvements. Recognising and valuing good practice and individual or collective initiatives that enhance safety helps to anchor this culture within the team.

Finally, a culture of safety goes hand in hand with a culture of continuous improvement. This implies regular questioning, adaptability in the face of new data and a constant desire to do better, for the well-being of the patient and the whole team.

Promoting a culture of safety in maxillo-facial surgery is an ongoing process, based on collaboration, training, accountability and open communication. By putting safety at the heart of everything we do, the team can offer the best possible care.

Breathe in and prepare the next generation of nurses

The future of healthcare rests on the shoulders of the next generation of medical professionals, and maxillofacial nurses have a vital role to play in this landscape. Inspiring and preparing this new wave of enthusiasts is a crucial mission, combining mentoring, education, practical experience and personal development.

To begin with, it is vital to show these future professionals the real and tangible impact they can have on patients' lives. Real-life stories, patient testimonials and feedback from experienced nurses can serve as concrete examples, showing not only the challenges of the profession but also the emotional rewards it offers.

Mentoring is a cornerstone of training. Having a guide, a confidant, someone who shares their knowledge and experience is invaluable to a young nurse. Mentors can help guide a career, develop clinical skills and navigate the emotional and ethical complexities of the profession.

Formal education remains, of course, at the heart of preparation. Training programmes must be continually updated to reflect medical advances, new technologies and current best practice. In addition, practical training, through internships and simulations, enables students to familiarise themselves with the real environment of an operating theatre or care unit.

Personal development is also essential. Maxillofacial surgery nurses are often faced with stressful, emotionally charged situations, and need to demonstrate resilience, empathy and communication skills. Workshops and training courses focusing on well-being, stress management and effective communication are all tools that will prepare these nurses to face the emotional challenges of their profession.

To inspire, we also need to show the diversity of opportunities. Maxillofacial surgery, although specialised, offers a multitude of career paths, whether in research, education, management or specialist clinical practice.

Finally, it is important to cultivate a sense of belonging to a community. Encouraging participation in professional associations, conferences and networking events gives young nurses a broader vision of their role and connects them to a close-knit, supportive community.

Preparing the next generation of maxillofacial surgery nurses means investing in the future of healthcare, ensuring quality care for patients and continuing to drive forward this exciting specialty. It's a shared responsibility, requiring dedication, passion and a vision for the future.

Chapter 28:
MANAGEMENT OF SPECIFIC CASES

Maxillo-facial surgery
in the elderly

With increasing life expectancy and a better understanding of the specific health needs of the elderly, maxillofacial surgery in this population has become an increasingly relevant topic. The surgical approach to elderly patients presents unique challenges and opportunities, requiring careful attention to clinical, physiological and psychosocial details.

The elderly are often faced with complex medical issues. Their bodies have undergone decades of wear and tear, exposure to various diseases and physiological changes that can influence the way they react to surgery. Co-morbidities, such as heart disease, diabetes or hypertension, are common and can complicate pre-, intra- and post-operative management.

The ageing process also directly affects the maxillofacial region. Bones may become more fragile or resorb, tissues lose elasticity and skin thins. These changes can influence the type of procedure recommended and the expectations for results.

The psychosocial aspect should not be neglected. Elderly patients may have concerns about their appearance, identity and quality of life post-operatively. It is essential to recognise and respect these concerns, while providing appropriate education and emotional support.

Communicating with elderly patients often requires a tailored approach. There may be barriers related to hearing or cognitive deficits, or simply increased anxiety about the procedure. Establishing a relationship of trust is vital, as is ensuring that the patient and their family are fully informed and comfortable with the proposed treatment plan.

The recovery period can also be prolonged or more complex in the elderly. It is crucial to anticipate and manage potential complications, ensure regular follow-up and provide rehabilitation tailored to their specific needs.

Working closely with other specialists, such as geriatricians, cardiologists or anaesthetists, is often essential to ensure complete and safe care. These multidisciplinary teams make it possible to tackle the specific challenges of elderly patients from every angle.

Maxillofacial surgery on the elderly is a rich and complex speciality. It requires medical expertise, a deep understanding of age-related changes and a humane, empathetic approach. The rewards, however, are immense, as it offers this population the opportunity to improve their quality of life, self-esteem and general health.

Patient care with specific needs (disability, co-morbidities)

Maxillofacial surgery, like other medical specialities, requires an individualised approach, especially when it comes to treating patients with specific needs. These patients may have physical or mental disabilities, co-morbidities or other particularities that make their care both delicate and essential.

A patient with a disability, whether visible such as a motor impairment, or invisible such as an autistic spectrum disorder, requires special consideration. It is essential to ensure easy access to facilities, to adjust equipment if necessary, but also to adapt communication to ensure the patient's understanding and comfort. Simple measures, such as the presence of a sign language interpreter or the use of visual aids, can make all the difference.

Co-morbidities add another layer of complexity. A patient with diabetes, for example, may have difficulty healing, while a patient with cardiovascular disease may have increased risks associated with anaesthesia. Collaboration with other specialists, such as endocrinologists, cardiologists or nephrologists, is often necessary to develop a safe and effective treatment plan.

Ongoing training of medical and paramedical staff is essential to ensure that they are well equipped to meet the needs of these patients. This includes not only medical training, but also training in communication, psychology and sociology to better understand and respond to patients' needs.

The key is active listening and compassion. It is essential to recognise and validate each patient's concerns and needs, and to strive to provide patient-centred care that takes into account the totality of the patient's being.

Technology also plays a major role. The use of adapted equipment, specialised applications to facilitate communication or innovative surgical techniques can greatly improve the quality of care provided.

Caring for patients with special needs in maxillofacial surgery is not just a question of medical competence. It is a holistic approach that requires empathy, interdisciplinarity and a constant desire to adapt and improve care to meet the needs of each individual.

Patients with a previous history surgery or treatment

A patient's surgical or treatment history is often crucial when planning and carrying out maxillofacial surgery procedures. Accurate knowledge of this history helps not only to anticipate potential challenges, but also to prevent potential complications.

When a patient has undergone previous surgery in the maxillofacial region, this may mean that anatomical structures have been modified or even altered. For example, tissue scars may limit the elasticity of the skin or obstruct access to certain areas. Similarly, pre-existing bone grafts or implants may influence the way in which a new operation is planned and carried out.

In addition, patients who have undergone treatments such as radiotherapy may have altered tissues that heal differently and are more susceptible to infection. Radiotherapy, particularly in the head and neck region, can lead to a reduction in tissue vascularisation, making irradiated areas more vulnerable.

It is also essential to take into account any medication that the patient may have taken or is still taking, as these can influence the response to anaesthesia, blood coagulation and the ability to heal. For example, patients on anticoagulants may require specific management to minimise the risk of bleeding.

Dialogue with the patient is essential to obtain a complete medical history. Previous medical records, X-ray images, operative reports and any other relevant documents must be carefully examined.

Interdisciplinary collaboration with other specialists who have treated the patient in the past is also beneficial. They can provide valuable information on the nature and results of previous interventions or treatments, as well as recommendations for the next steps.

Managing a patient with a history of maxillofacial surgery or treatment requires a meticulous, informed and collaborative approach. Every patient is unique, and the history of their health and previous treatments is an essential chapter in guaranteeing optimal and safe care for future operations.

Chapter 29:
MAXILLO-FACIAL SURGERY
IN A GLOBAL CONTEXT

Differences and similarities in care around the world

Maxillofacial surgery, although rooted in universal medical principles, is influenced by a variety of factors around the world, including cultural, socio-economic and educational factors. That said, while recognising these variations, it is essential to note that there are also striking similarities in the approach to this specialty.

Similarities:
- **Fundamental principles**: The anatomical and physiological principles that guide maxillofacial surgery are universal. Bone, muscle, vascular and nerve structures are consistent from one individual to another, regardless of location.
- **Treatment objectives**: Regardless of the context, the main aim of maxillofacial surgery is to restore form and function, while ensuring the patient's well-being.
- **Education and training**: Although training pathways may vary, the emphasis is generally on solid academic and clinical training. Many institutions strive to meet international standards.

The differences:
- **Access to care**: In developed countries, access to maxillofacial surgical care is often more readily available thanks to robust healthcare infrastructures. However, in some developing regions, access may be limited due to financial or geographical constraints, or a shortage of specialists.

- **Technologies and equipment** : Advanced technologies, such as robot-assisted surgery and 3D imaging, are widely available in wealthy countries. On the other hand, these innovations may be out of reach or limited in less privileged regions.
- **Cultural and social practices**: Aesthetic standards, religious beliefs and cultural traditions can influence the demand for specific procedures and how they are perceived. For example, in some cultures a scar may be considered a sign of bravery, while in others it may be seen as stigmatising.
- **Regulations and standards**: Clinical standards, treatment protocols and regulatory requirements may vary considerably from one country to another.

Although maxillofacial surgery is based on universal principles, the application and practice of this specialty often reflect the complex mix of cultural, economic and educational influences specific to each region of the world. However, with globalisation and the increased sharing of knowledge, there is a growing convergence of standards and practices, promoting a better quality of care for all.

Contributing to international medical missions

International medical missions represent an opportunity for healthcare professionals to transcend borders, provide care to those who need it most and learn from different cultures and environments. These missions can take many forms, from responding to natural disasters to reconstructive surgery and vaccination programmes. Here's how an individual can contribute to these vital missions:

- **Assessing your skills**: Before taking the plunge, it's crucial to assess your skills and experience. Some may offer surgical expertise, while others may have skills in health education or logistics.
- **Research and selection of credible organisations**: There are many non-governmental organisations (NGOs) and associations that organise medical missions. It is essential to choose a reputable organisation with a proven track record for quality care and ethics.
- **Training and preparation**: It is often necessary to undergo specific training before leaving. This may include courses in tropical health, emergency response, local culture or language.
- **Flexibility and adaptability**: Working in conditions that differ from those in your usual practice requires a high degree of adaptability. Resources may be limited and protocols may vary.
- **Intercultural collaboration**: Respect for and understanding of local customs, beliefs and traditions are essential to establishing a relationship of trust with the local community and other team members.
- **Long-term commitment**: Although some missions are of short duration, it can be beneficial to make a longer-term commitment to ensure continuity of care and the training of local professionals.
- **Sharing and education**: On their return, participants can share their experiences with colleagues, offering a unique perspective and raising awareness of the importance of comprehensive care.
- **Financial or in-kind support**: If you can't physically take part in a mission, you can still support these initiatives by making financial donations, providing medical equipment or taking part in fundraising events.
- **Emotional preparation**: Medical missions can be both rewarding and emotionally demanding. It is

crucial to be mentally prepared and to have support mechanisms in place.
- **Ethical standards**: It is imperative to maintain the highest ethical standards, always acting in the best interests of patients.

Contributing to international medical missions is an enriching experience that not only offers the opportunity to help others, but also to learn, grow and see the world in a different light. With passion and commitment, every individual can make a significant difference.

Understanding care disparities and remedies

Disparities in care are unequal and unfair differences in health and health provision between different population groups. These disparities can be based on a multitude of factors, including race, ethnicity, gender, age, socio-economic level, sexual orientation, geography and other socio-demographic characteristics. Understanding and remedying these disparities is crucial to ensuring equal care for all.

1. Acknowledging the existence of disparities :
It is essential to recognise that disparities exist. Studies and research clearly show that certain groups receive inferior healthcare because of prejudice, stereotypes and systemic barriers.

2. Education and training :
Raising awareness and educating medical staff and healthcare providers about existing disparities and their causes can help reduce unconscious prejudice. Cultural training can help healthcare professionals understand the specific needs of patients from different backgrounds.

3. Access to healthcare :
Disparities are often linked to accessibility. It is essential to ensure that everyone has access to quality care, whether this means making services available in rural areas, reducing costs for people on low incomes or providing language services for non-English speakers.

4. Community involvement :
Listening to and working directly with affected communities to understand their needs and co-create solutions. This can also help build trust between healthcare providers and communities.

5. Data collection and analysis :
It is crucial to collect data on race, ethnicity, language and other socio-demographic indicators. This data can be used to identify where disparities exist and monitor progress in closing them.

6. Oriented search :
Promote research focusing on the health of minority populations and health disparities. This can help develop specific interventions and inform public policy.

7. Cross-sector collaboration :
Work with other sectors, such as education, housing, employment and transport, to tackle the social determinants of health that contribute to disparities.

8. Advocacy :
Healthcare professionals and institutions can play a leading role in advocating equitable policies, whether at local, national or international level.

9. Resources and funding :
Allocate resources and funding specifically to address health disparities. This may include grants for research, community programmes or educational initiatives.

10. Continuous assessment :
Regular monitoring and evaluation of progress is essential to ensure that disparities are genuinely reduced.

Remedying disparities in care requires a concerted, multi-dimensional effort on the part of all stakeholders in the healthcare sector. Every step taken to reduce these inequalities brings society closer to achieving a truly equitable healthcare system for all.

Chapter 30:
ETHICAL ISSUES
AND SOCIETAL ADVANCES

Managing cases where the patient's expectations differ from medical advice

When a patient's expectations diverge from medical advice or recommendations, this can lead to complex and delicate situations. It is essential to approach these differences with sensitivity, respect and professionalism. Here is an approach for navigating these situations:

1. Active listening :
Always start by listening to the patient, without interrupting. Understanding where the patient is coming from, their fears, concerns and expectations is fundamental to establishing a dialogue.
2. Ask open-ended questions:
Encourage discussion by asking questions that encourage the patient to express their feelings, concerns and wishes, such as "Can you tell me more about your concerns?"
3. Validate the patient's feelings:
Even if you don't agree, it's crucial to validate the patient's feelings. You might say, "I understand why you might feel that way..."
4. Clarify your recommendations:
Restate your professional views clearly and simply and explain the underlying reasons for your recommendation. Use evidence and data to support your opinion.
5. Address concerns and myths:
The patient may have misinformation or preconceived ideas. Tactfully address these points, providing clear, factual information.

6. Explain the risks and benefits:
Make sure the patient understands the advantages and disadvantages, risks and benefits of each option.

7. Offer alternatives, if possible :
If medically appropriate, discuss alternatives or compromises that might satisfy both the patient and medical standards.

8. Encourage a second opinion:
If the patient remains hesitant or unsure, suggest they get a second opinion. This can increase the patient's confidence in the decision-making process.

9. Ensure that the patient gives informed consent:
If the patient decides to take a different route from your recommendation, make sure they understand the implications of their decision and document it.

10. Document the conversation:
Take detailed notes of what was discussed, including the patient's concerns and recommendations given.

11. Follow-up:
Offer to follow up with the patient after a period of time to see how they are doing and discuss any further concerns.

12. Think about your own communication:
It's always good to reflect on how you communicate with patients. Look for ways to continually improve to make communication as clear and empathetic as possible.

Managing these differences requires a combination of empathy, listening, education and collaboration. The aim is to ensure that patients receive appropriate care while respecting their autonomy and personal choices.

Medical decisions in specific cultural or religious contexts

Navigating the medical landscape requires a deep sensitivity and understanding of patients' cultural and religious backgrounds. These beliefs and practices can influence how patients perceive illness, treatment, death and the role of healthcare professionals. Here is a fluid exploration of the challenges and recommended approaches in these situations:

The world is a complex mosaic of cultures, traditions and beliefs. Each culture and religion brings with it a rich tapestry of rituals, practices and values that can often play a dominant role in the way people approach their healthcare.

Imagine a Muslim patient who, during the holy month of Ramadan, chooses to fast from sunrise to sunset. This decision could have implications for the administration of medication, the management of blood sugar levels or even the scheduling of surgery. Or consider Jehovah's Witnesses, whose beliefs prohibit blood transfusions, posing unique challenges in surgery or oncology.

For the healthcare professional, the first step is to recognise and validate these differences. Empathy is the key. It's not just about understanding what the patient is feeling, but also why they are feeling it. Taking the time to ask questions, listen carefully and create a space where the patient feels respected and heard is crucial.

But listening is only half the equation. Education also plays an essential role. In some cases, it may be possible to find a compromise that respects the patient's beliefs while guaranteeing their safety. For example, could medication schedules be reorganised during Ramadan, or alternatives to blood transfusions be used for Jehovah's Witnesses?

There are also times when medicine and cultural or religious beliefs may come into direct conflict. In such cases, clear, honest and respectful communication is essential. It is important to ensure that the patient (or their family) fully understands the risks and benefits associated with each decision.

Working with community or religious leaders can also be beneficial. These individuals can offer valuable insights, help mediate and provide spiritual support to the patient.

Making medical decisions in specific cultural or religious contexts is a delicate balancing act. It requires flexibility, patience, respect and, above all, humility. In this balancing act, it is essential to remember that each patient is unique, with his or her own history, beliefs and needs. And it is by recognising and honouring this individuality that healthcare professionals can offer the best possible care.

The ethics of cosmetic surgery for non-medical purposes

Cosmetic surgery, a branch of plastic surgery, has long been the subject of ethical debate, particularly when practised for non-medical purposes. The rise of cosmetic surgery in a world where appearance plays a key role highlights complex questions about individual autonomy, identity, societal pressures and the limits of medicine.

Join me on a journey through the nuanced world of ethical reflection:
At the heart of the debate is the idea of autonomy. Do individuals have the right to modify their bodies as they see fit, even if this is not medically necessary? Most ethicists would argue that yes, adults have the right to make informed decisions about their own bodies, as long as it does not harm others.

But here, the word "informed" takes on vital importance. Informed consent is not just about understanding the medical risks, but also about being aware of underlying motivations, potentially unrealistic expectations, and the influence of societal norms. If a person wishes to undergo an operation because of social pressure or low self-esteem, is the decision truly autonomous?

Which brings us to another crucial point: aesthetic standards are, to a large extent, shaped by culture, society and the media. In a society obsessed with youth and beauty, can we say that the desire for an intervention is truly a free choice, or is it the product of external influences and often unattainable standards?
There is also the question of resources. In many parts of the world, access to medical care is limited. Is it ethical to use precious medical resources for non-essential cosmetic procedures, when others could benefit from vital medical care?

And then there's the commercial aspect. Cosmetic surgery is a lucrative industry. How can we be sure that the decisions taken by surgeons are not influenced by financial gain? Are patients being exploited, or is cosmetic surgery simply a response to legitimate market demand?

Finally, there is the debate about the very essence of medicine. The Hippocratic Oath states: "First, do no harm". But what does 'harm' mean in this context? If an intervention improves a person's psychological well-being, even if it is not medically necessary, can it be said to be harmful?

Navigating these ethical waters requires deep reflection, not only on the part of surgeons themselves, but also on the part of society as a whole. As cosmetic surgery continues to evolve, it is imperative that the ethical debate evolves too, with a focus on the well-being, autonomy and dignity of each individual.

Chapter 31:
FUTURE PROSPECTS AND VISION

The challenges ahead
for maxillo-facial surgery

Maxillofacial surgery, while evolving rapidly with significant technological advances, faces a number of future challenges. Let's take a closer look at some of these challenges and the associated prospects.

1. Adapting to new technologies :
   * **Challenge:** Advances such as robot-assisted surgery and 3D printing offer new possibilities, but also require constant training and adaptation on the part of surgeons.
   * **Outlook:** Training and certification programmes will have to evolve to incorporate these skills, ensuring that surgeons are not only technically competent but also capable of making full use of the technological tools available.
2. Management of Patients with Complex Conditions :
   * **Challenge:** Managing patients with complex co-morbidities, such as the elderly or those with chronic illnesses, requires a multidisciplinary approach.
   * **Outlook:** Closer collaboration with other medical specialities and an emphasis on a holistic approach to care are essential.
3. Access to surgical care :
   * **Challenge:** Many patients around the world do not have access to basic surgical care, a problem exacerbated in low-resource regions.
   * **Outlook:** Maxillo-facial surgeons and professional organisations must advocate for a better distribution

of resources and work to improve access to care in under-serviced areas.

4. Managing Patients' Expectations :
   - **Challenge:** With the increase in aesthetic procedures, managing patient expectations is becoming increasingly crucial.
   - **Perspective:** Clear, honest communication and patient education on possible outcomes and risks are fundamental.

5. Ethical issues :
   - **Challenge:** Ethical issues, particularly concerning non-essential cosmetic surgery, require careful thought and navigation.
   - **Perspective:** An ongoing commitment to fundamental ethical principles and an open and honest discussion of these issues are imperative.

6. Research and Development :
   - **Challenge:** Maxillo-facial surgery research must continue to progress in order to improve surgical techniques and patient outcomes.
   - **Outlook:** Increased investment in research and development is essential if the specialty is to move forward.

7. Training and Education :
   - **Challenge:** Ensuring high-quality continuing education and training for maxillo-facial surgeons is essential.
   - **Perspective:** Educational institutions and hospitals must commit to providing high-quality continuing education and training opportunities.
   -

While maxillofacial surgery faces these and other challenges, proactively addressing these issues and adopting innovations can help the specialty move forward, improving care and outcomes for patients worldwide.

The future of nursing training in this speciality

The future of nursing education, particularly in the specialty of maxillofacial surgery, promises to be both dynamic and constantly evolving. Let's take a look at the main trends, innovations and adaptations we can expect to see:

1. Simulation-based training :
Simulation technologies have grown rapidly. The training of nurses in this speciality is expected to include more and more simulation sessions, providing a safe environment to practise advanced skills before interacting with real patients.

2. Continuing Education and Specialisation :
With the rapid evolution of medical technology and surgical techniques, nurses will need to engage in continuing education to stay up to date. Advanced training modules or specialist certifications could be offered.

3. Multidisciplinary approach :
The importance of team-centred patient care will be reinforced. Training will encourage greater collaboration between nurses, surgeons, anaesthetists, speech therapists and other healthcare professionals.
4. Focus on soft skills :
In addition to clinical skills, greater emphasis will be placed on training in communication, empathy, stress management and ethical decision-making.

5. Technology and telemedicine :
The future is likely to see greater incorporation of technology into nursing care. Nurses will be trained to use telemedicine tools, patient monitoring applications and other emerging technologies.

6. Cultural and ethical training :
The training will emphasise the importance of understanding the diverse cultural, religious and individual perspectives of patients, and how these can influence care.

7. Research and Participation in Evidence-Based Practice :
Nurses will be encouraged to participate in clinical research and to apply practices based on solid evidence, thereby improving standards of care.

8. Hybrid learning :
With the development of e-learning technologies, we can expect a combination of traditional classroom learning and e-learning, offering students greater flexibility.

9. Diversified clinical investments :
Internship opportunities could extend beyond traditional hospital centres to include specialist clinics, medical missions abroad and ambulatory care centres.

10. Strengthening management skills :
With the potential for advanced and leadership roles for specialist nurses, modules on team management, administration and resource management could be integrated.

The future of nursing education in maxillofacial surgery promises to be rich and varied, adapting nurses to the changing needs of patients and the evolving global medical landscape. These adaptations will ensure high-quality care, while providing nurses with the skills they need to thrive in their specialist careers.

Vision and aspirations for optimum care

In an ever-changing world, where medicine and technology are advancing at breakneck speed, the ideal of optimal care can seem like a moving target. Nevertheless, our vision of optimal care is rooted in timeless principles, while embracing innovation and adaptability. Here's an outline of that vision, and the aspirations that underpin each element:

1. Patient-centred :
Every patient is unique, with individual needs, values and aspirations. Optimal care recognises and honours this uniqueness, putting the patient at the centre of all medical decisions.

2. Holistic approach :
Care should not be limited to treating an illness or a symptom. It must embrace all facets of the individual: physical, mental, emotional, social and spiritual.

3. Universal Access :
Everyone, whatever their origins, financial situation or geographical location, should have access to quality healthcare.

4. Integration of Advanced Technologies :
Although technology alone cannot define optimal care, it can make a major contribution. The integration of medical innovations, telemedicine and other technological tools will improve diagnosis, treatment and follow-up.

5. Continuing education :
Healthcare professionals must engage in continuous learning, ensuring that their skills and knowledge reflect current best practice.

6. Transparent and Effective Communication :
Clear communication between patients, their families and healthcare professionals is crucial. It builds trust, improves compliance with treatment and encourages informed decision-making.

7. Collaborative Decision Making :
Patients must take responsibility for their own health, working closely with their healthcare providers in the decision-making process.

8. Research and Innovation :
Optimal care requires constant exploration of new methods, treatments and approaches, supported by rigorous research.

9. Safety :
Ensuring patient safety is paramount, with clear protocols to minimise errors and manage complications effectively.
10. Ethics and Integrity :
All care must be provided with respect for human dignity, with strict adherence to high ethical standards.

Our aspiration is simple: to offer every patient the best possible care, in an environment of compassion, excellence, innovation and respect. By always keeping this vision in mind, we can navigate through the challenges of the modern medical world, while providing care that truly elevates the human condition.

Chapter 32:
PRACTICAL ADVICE AND RESOURCES

Managing stress
and burnout

Managing stress and burnout is a major concern in many professional fields, particularly those related to health. The intensity of responsibilities, long working hours and emotionally charged situations can quickly lead to a feeling of burnout. Recognising the warning signs and implementing proactive strategies can help prevent and deal with these challenges.

Symptoms :
Burnout doesn't happen overnight. It sets in gradually and manifests itself through various symptoms:
- **Physical:** Persistent fatigue, trouble sleeping, headaches or muscle pain.
- **Emotional:** Feelings of isolation, dejection, cynicism or increased irritability.
- **Behavioural:** Reduced productivity, avoidance of work, changes in eating or drinking habits.

Management strategies :
- **Setting limits: It'**s essential to know how to say no and to define clear boundaries between work and personal life. This can mean disconnecting work emails outside working hours or taking regular breaks during the day.
- **Taking care of yourself:** Activities such as meditation, yoga, physical exercise and a balanced diet can help manage stress.
- **Social Connection:** Talking to colleagues, friends or a therapist can provide emotional support. Solidarity

and sharing experiences can offer perspective and relief.

- **Pursuing a passion:** Having a hobby or activity outside work can help you relax and disconnect from work pressures.
- **Education and training:** Taking part in training courses on stress management or resilience can provide tools for managing difficult situations.
- **Take a holiday:** Taking regular time out to rest and recharge is vital for preventing burnout.
- **Seek help:** If the stress becomes overwhelming, it may be helpful to consult a health professional, such as a psychologist or counsellor.
- **Reconsider Role or Career:** In certain cases, a transition to another position or another speciality may be necessary to preserve mental and emotional health.
- **Organisational culture:** Employers also have a role to play in creating a healthy working environment, recognising the signs of burnout in employees and offering appropriate support.

Managing stress and burnout requires a proactive approach from both individuals and organisations. By paying attention to the warning signs and taking preventive measures, it is possible to maintain a healthy work-life balance.

Keeping up to date advances in the field

Keeping abreast of advances in a professional field, especially one as dynamic as maxillofacial medicine and surgery, is absolutely crucial. Adapting to innovations and new methodologies is essential to provide the best possible patient care, to remain competitive and to continue to develop as a professional. Here are some tips on how to keep up to date:

- **Subscriptions to Scientific Journals:** There are many academic journals that regularly publish articles based on recent research. These journals are often the first place where new discoveries are shared with the medical community.
- **Conferences and Seminars:** Attending professional conferences allows you not only to hear about the latest research directly from the experts, but also to network with other professionals and share experiences.
- **Continuing education:** Many health-related professions have continuing education requirements. This can take the form of online courses, workshops or practical sessions.
- **Online communities and forums:** There are countless online forums and groups where professionals can ask questions, share discoveries or discuss the latest news in their field.
- **Books and Publications:** In addition to scientific journals, many experts publish books that explore certain subjects in greater depth or present new perspectives.
- **Networking:** Talking to colleagues, taking part in discussion groups and joining professional associations can offer many opportunities to learn from others.
- **Technology:** Use applications, software or other technological tools designed specifically for your field. These are often updated with the latest knowledge and may offer integrated training or tutorials.
- **Universities and research institutions:** Working with academic institutions can provide access to cutting-edge research, clinical trials and other valuable resources.

- **Check out Specialist Media:** Some websites, YouTube channels, podcasts or blogs are dedicated to disseminating the latest news and trends in specific fields.
- **Adopt a Continuous Learning Mentality:** A proactive attitude to learning is essential. Instead of waiting for information to come to you, actively seek out new knowledge and be open to change.

Keeping up to date requires an active commitment. Medicine is a constantly evolving field, with new discoveries, techniques and technologies emerging frequently. By investing time and effort in keeping up to date, professionals can offer their patients a better quality of care and enrich their own careers.

Resources and professional associations

Professional resources and associations play a fundamental role in supporting healthcare professionals, particularly those involved in maxillofacial surgery. These organisations offer opportunities for continuing education, networking and access to cutting-edge research, and they often represent the interests of their members to government institutions and the public.

- Professional Associations :
  - **International Association of Oral and Maxillofacial Surgeons (IAOMS)**: This is one of the leading organisations dedicated to oral and maxillofacial surgery. It promotes the exchange of knowledge and resources between surgeons worldwide.
  - **American Association of Oral and Maxillofacial Surgeons (AAOMS)**: For professionals based in the United States, the

AAOMS offers training, conferences and relevant publications.
- Other countries often have their own national associations specifically for maxillofacial surgery.
- Newspapers and Magazines :
    - **Journal of Oral and Maxillofacial Surgery (JOMS)**: A leading journal in the field, publishing articles based on recent research.
    - **International Journal of Oral and Maxillofacial Surgery**: Another important source for the latest research and case studies.
- **Conferences and Seminars:** These events are essential for networking, learning the latest techniques and discovering new research. The associations mentioned above regularly organise conferences.
- **Online training:** Many websites, universities and associations offer online courses to help professionals keep abreast of the latest techniques and discoveries.
- **Forums and Discussion Groups:** These platforms enable professionals to exchange ideas, ask questions and share experiences with their peers from around the world.
- Other resources :
    - **Medical libraries and databases**: Resources such as PubMed offer access to a vast collection of articles and research.
    - **Certification bodies**: These institutions establish and maintain professional standards. They often offer resources to help professionals obtain and renew their certification.
- **Interprofessional collaboration:** Linking up with associations in related fields, such as dentistry, plastic surgery, oncology, etc., can offer broader perspectives and opportunities for collaboration.

To maximise the benefits of these resources, professionals are advised to get actively involved: join associations, attend conferences, take part in discussions, and keep up to date with publications in leading journals. These steps not only ensure informed practice, but also strengthen the professional's reputation and credibility in his or her community.

Chapter 33:
CONCLUSION
TOWARDS A PROMISING FUTURE

The invaluable contribution of the maxillo-facial surgery nurse

Maxillofacial surgery, with its complex range of procedures from the correction of congenital malformations to post-traumatic reconstruction, requires specialised expertise not only from the surgeon, but also from the entire medical team. At the heart of this team, the maxillofacial surgery nurse makes an invaluable contribution.

A patient's first interaction with a nurse can determine the tone of the surgical experience. Through their empathetic approach, nurses reassure patients and their families, clarify their doubts and establish a climate of trust. They play an essential role in pre-operative preparation, ensuring that the patient understands the procedure, its benefits and its risks.

During surgery, the operating theatre nurse works closely with the surgeon, anticipating his or her needs, ensuring sterility and safety, while constantly monitoring the patient's well-being. The nurse's speed, precision and skill can significantly influence the course of surgery.

The post-operative phase is just as crucial. The nurse monitors pain, watches for signs of complications, guides the patient through post-operative care, and often acts as a liaison between the patient, the family and the medical team. The nurse's ability to teach, reassure and encourage can speed up recovery and optimise surgical results.

But beyond technical skills, it is perhaps in the emotional realm that nurses shine brightest. Maxillofacial surgery can often have a profound impact on a patient's identity and self-esteem, and the psychological support offered by the nurse is vital. Whether it's listening to a patient's concerns, sharing post-operative successes or guiding a patient through the challenges of rehabilitation, the nurse is often the emotional lifeline that the patient leans on.

Maxillo-facial surgery nurses also contribute to continuing education, research, protocol improvement and policy development. Because of their proximity to the patient, they are often the first to identify areas for improvement, proposing innovative solutions to improve care and efficiency.

The value of the maxillofacial surgery nurse lies in their ability to fuse technical skill, compassionate care and clinical expertise to deliver a holistic patient experience. In a field where every millimetre counts, where function and form meet, and where the physical and emotional are inextricably linked, the nurse stands out as a central pillar of the surgical experience.

The impact of technology and innovation for the future

The impact of technology and innovation on the future is a wide-ranging subject that affects almost every area of our lives. In medicine, communications, education, industry and even our everyday lives, technology and innovation are the catalysts shaping the future.

1. Medicine and healthcare :
Telemedicine, robot-assisted surgery, genomics and artificial intelligence in diagnostics are radically

transforming healthcare. Diseases that were once incurable are now treatable thanks to gene therapy. Medical wearables enable continuous monitoring, providing valuable data for early diagnosis and prevention.

2. Communications :
5G and future technologies promise faster communication speeds, reduced latency, and ubiquitous connectivity. This facilitates the rise of smart cities, connected vehicles and the Internet of Things (IoT).

3. Education :
Virtual and augmented reality, e-learning platforms and AI are personalising the educational experience, making learning more accessible and tailored to learners' individual needs.

4. Energy and the environment :
Innovations in renewable energies, such as solar and wind power, as well as advances in energy storage, are pointing towards a greener future. Carbon capture and storage technologies could also play a crucial role in the fight against climate change.

5. Industry and manufacturing :
3D printing, advanced robotics and the Industrial Internet of Things are revolutionising production, enabling more agile, customised and local manufacturing.

6. Economics and finance :
Cryptocurrencies, blockchain and fintechs are redefining transactions, trust and security in the financial world.

7. Daily :
From home automation to augmented reality for shopping, technology is improving and simplifying our daily lives.

However, with this progress come challenges. Questions of confidentiality, ethics, security and fairness are becoming increasingly acute. For example, how do we ensure that AI, in its automatic learning, does not incorporate bias? How do companies regulate and adopt new technologies without stifling innovation?

The future, with the help of technology and innovation, is full of promise, but it also requires careful thought, judicious regulation and responsible adoption to ensure that these advances benefit everyone fairly.

Inspire the next generation of nurses

Inspiring the next generation of nurses is more than a question of technical training. It is also, and perhaps above all, a question of igniting an inner flame, of passing on passion and values. Nurses are at the heart of the care-giver-patient relationship, and embody both the science and the humanity of the medical profession.

1. Stories and testimonials :
Real-life stories, successes and challenges overcome can be a major source of inspiration. The new generation needs to hear the stories of those who have been on the front line during health crises, who have accompanied patients at the end of their lives or who have experienced incredible moments of hope.
2. The human dimension :
Stressing the human impact of the nursing role is essential. The simple act of holding a patient's hand, reassuring a family or offering a smile can have an enormous impact. This human connection, this deep bond that is created between nurse and patient, is unique and should be valued.

3. Innovative training :

Learning techniques are evolving. Simulations, virtual reality and interactive case studies can make training more dynamic and closer to real-life situations.

4. Mentoring :

Setting up mentoring programmes can help young nurses to project themselves into their future role. Having a mentor, someone to guide, advise and share experiences with, can be a determining factor in a young professional's vocation.

5. Promoting the profession :

It is crucial to enhance the role of nurses in the healthcare system. This requires recognition in terms of both salary and social status. A well-regarded and respected nurse will inspire more vocations.

6. Adaptability:

The world of healthcare is changing rapidly. The next generation of nurses must be prepared to adapt, learn and evolve throughout their careers. This means promoting continuous training and encouraging professional curiosity.

7. Social commitment:

The new generation is increasingly socially committed. The social and ethical dimension of the nursing profession needs to be highlighted. Taking part in humanitarian missions, getting involved in causes or defending patients' rights are all aspects that can be attractive and inspiring.

Finally, every nurse, through their dedication, professionalism and passion, is already a source of inspiration. It's important to give everyone the means to share their experience, pass on their knowledge and embody the core values of this vital profession.

www.ingramcontent.com/pod-product-compliance
Lightning Source LLC
Chambersburg PA
CBHW072155290526
45794CB00004B/1514